ECONOMIC COMMISSION FOR EUROPE
Geneva

DIGITAL IMAGING IN HEALTH CARE

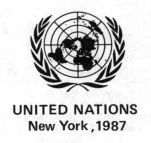

UNITED NATIONS
New York , 1987

ECE/ENG.AUT/25

UNITED NATIONS PUBLICATION

Sales No. E.86.II.E.29

ISBN 92-1-116380-3

04800P

CONTENTS

GE.86-24473/6441E, 6446E,
6452E and 6454E

LIST OF TABLES

Chapter III

Chapter IV

Chapter V

LIST OF FIGURES

The United Nations Economic Commission for Europe (ECE) - established 40 years ago - has from the outset recognized the major role of engineering industries in general industrial development.

The engineering industries, as dominant producers and suppliers of machinery and equipment to all other economic sectors, constitute the core of the economy and reflect the overall economic climate. It is therefore quite natural that the Commission should allocate increasing importance to the techno-economic studies, seminars, statistical reviews and other work being undertaken by its Working Party on Engineering Industries and Automation.

ECE member countries (all European countries, United States and Canada) have long recognized the need to improve quality and reliaiblity and labour and capital productivity in manufacturing industries. New approaches towards automation of engineering technologies, development of new materials, design of products with new qualitative attributes and computerization of management and control functions have also significantly contributed to lowering production costs and improving product competitiveness.

The Working Party has carried out several important projects in the area of information technology, covering such topics as industrial robotics, flexible manufacturing systems, telecommunication equipment or software tools. Systematic efforts also continue in the study of developments in other traditional engineering sectors in order to analyse the significant techno-economic impact and associated social implications of major technological developments affecting the ongoing process of restructuring.

The annexed list (see annex I) of 21 seminars held since 1971 under the auspices of the Working Party and its predecessors, the Working Party on Automation and the ad hoc Meeting of Experts on Engineering Industries, illustrates the wide scope of selected themes, including, as from 1983, the important field of biomedical engineering.

During the last decade, the electrical and electronic engineering sector, particularly affected by the revolutionary developments in microelectronics, showed the largest annual growth rates regarding both production and international trade. An important share in this respect belongs to biomedical engineering, which is marked by significant developments in electromedical equipment, especially digital imaging (generation, processing and recording of images). Computed tomography, magnetic resonance imaging, positron emission tomography, ultrasonic imaging and picture archiving and communication systems are no more a vision of tomorrow, but proved technologies and products increasingly applied in medical practice and significantly contributing to the improvement of the level of health care in the ECE region. In order to explain the main reasons which led to the inclusion of a study on digital imaging in health care in the programme of work of the Working Party, it might be useful briefly to recall the professional and organizational climate in which the study was created.

The Seminar on Innovation in Biomedical Equipment was held under the auspices of the Working Party at the invitation of the Goverment of Hungary in Budapest from 2 to 6 May 1983. Participants from 15 countries and 7 international organizations took part in the Seminar. A total of 45 papers were presented in four sections:

- Interaction between health care and the development of engineering products for biomedical purposes;

- Innovation trends in the health-related services and industries;

- Advanced biomedical equipment and systems; and

- International co-operation and trade and other factors influencing the development of biomedical equipment.

During the adoption of the Report of the Seminar, many significant conclusions were drawn and recommendations made. In particular "it was hoped that ECE activities of this type would continue and that there would be a follow-up to the results already achieved in this field ... Keeping in mind the wide use of biomedical equipment, which influenced daily life and could be instrumental in improving its quality while having a direct impact on the economies of countries, the participants felt that the Seminar had helped in pinpointing the socio-techno-economic consequences of the introduction of this equipment ... They felt that further study would be needed to understand better the influence of innovation on different types of biomedical equipment ...". [1]

The Working Party, at its fourth session, in March 1984, on the basis of proposals presented by the delegations of Hungary and Sweden and by the representative of the International Federation for Medical and Biological Engineering (IFMBE), decided to undertake a study on digital image processing as a follow-up to the Seminar held in 1983. The first ad hoc Meeting for the study was convened in November 1984. [2]

The subject of innovation in biomedical equipment covers a very broad area, both from the point of view of heterogeneity of equipment and different types and levels of innovation and the first ad hoc Meeting had the task of defining the precise scope and aim of the study. In this regard, the Meeting was expected to select a subject of common interest reflecting innovation in a high-technology area of health care which, at the same time, involved significant health-care expenditure in ECE countries. A preliminary draft outline for the study on innovation in biomedical equipment, emphasizing in particular the importance of digital image processing, was prepared by the secretariat. [3]

The participants in the first ad hoc Meeting agreed upon the selection of digital imaging (DI) as a significant topic illustrating recent trends in biomedical engineering. Mention was made of other leading-edge areas of development, such as intensive-care equipment (including cardiac monitoring), aids for the handicapped (including communication equipment) and new materials used in biology and medical sciences. It was, however, felt that DI should receive the highest priority and that the study of other topics could be considered subsequently if the work on DI proved to be of sufficient interest to ECE member countries. [4]

The fifth session of the Working Party, held in February/March 1985: [5]

- Approved the results of the first ad hoc Meeting and underlined that the topic of DI provided a good example of dynamic developments in health care closely related to other automation-oriented activities of the Working Party; and

- Requested the secretariat to proceed with the first draft of the study and to convene a second ad hoc Meeting to review the draft, in early 1986.

A circular letter to Governments and international organizations active in the field was sent out in February 1985, requesting:

- The nomination of experts who could act as rapporteurs and/or focal points for the study; and

- Contributions for individual chapters of the study, as well as other relevant material.

On the basis of contributions received from countries and international organizations active in the field and material from other available sources, a first draft of the principal part of the study was prepared in October 1985 by Professor N. Saranummi of the Technical Research Centre of Finland, Medical Engineering Laboratory at Tampere, an internationally renowned expert who is also associated with IFMBE.

The sixth session of the Working Party, held in March 1986, [6] after considering a progress report prepared by the secretariat, [7] decided to convene a second ad hoc Meeting for the study from 30 June to 2 July 1986 in order to overview the draft study and decide on the methods and timing of the finalization of the study, preferably before the end of 1986 so that it could be published in the form of an ECE sales publication early in 1987. */

---

*/   As a follow-up to the present study, the Working Party will organize a Seminar on Automation Means in Preventive Medicine '87, at Piestany, Czechoslovakia, from 28 September to 2 October 1987 - see Information Notice No. 1 for the Seminar. [9]

The Seminar will provide a forum for the exchange of information and experience in the field of preventive medical treatment, including the design, production and use of instruments, equipment and systems. Special emphasis will be put on various aspects of automation in diagnostic processes. Questions concerning techno-economic trends, international trade and other forms of co-operation, support programmes and relevant activities of international organizations, and various implementation and operational aspects, including the socio-economic impact of advanced medical equipment and systems for health care, will be discussed. The Seminar is expected to draw conclusions and make recommendations regarding future work which might be undertaken within the framework of the Working Party.

It is intended that the Seminar should adopt an interdisciplinary approach in order to bring together Government officials and directors and specialists from industrial enterprises and companies producing and supplying medical equipment, and from design and research institutes and universities, as well as main users, including physicians, hospital management and laboratory technologists, and foreign trade specialists. The Seminar is expected to further co-operation amongst medical engineering specialists and contribute to improving health-care systems and services.

The provisional programme for the Seminar and a list of suggested topics are presented in annex II.

The second _ad hoc_ Meeting [8] considered the draft study in detail and agreed on supplements, changes and modifications to the existing text. It also recommended that a simplified questionnaire should be issued to collect national contributions and the required statistical data. The title of the study was modified to read "Digital Imaging in Health Care". In the absence of similarly oriented studies, it was felt that the ECE study should:

- Address a broader audience than simply technicians directly involved in the introduction of DI technology;

- Include basic definitions and the principal technical characteristics of DI equipment and systems; and

- Clearly reflect the rising cost of health care and some other aspects of use such as peformance assurance.

When dealing with medical equipment, it was recognized that special attention should be paid to the need for an intersectoral approach, since the pace of innovation in this field is extremely rapid as regards the technologies and the application of equipment. Economic implications must be carefully considered before introducing new equipment. Health-care requirements grow and therefore need better-organized management systems.

The study of the field of medical engineering - and of digital imaging in particular - should be representative of the general trends in technologies, e.g. the increasing incorporation of microelectronic technology and computer hardware and software in equipment and systems. It should also reflect the interdependence of the social, economic, technical and organizational problems involved in the field.

Digital imaging is currently evolving rapidly owing to innovations both in imaging technologies and in technologies related to image handling. These changes will have a far-reaching effect on diagnostic services and on health care in general.

The "chain" consisting of the 1983 Budapest seminar - the current study on digital imaging - and the 1987 Piestany seminar forms a modest contribution of ECE to the ongoing process of innovation in biomedical equipment. It would have been impossible to undertake this responsible task without extensive support of well-known institutions and enthusiastic experts in many ECE member countries and without the benefit of the material provided by numerous international organizations active in the field (see table VII.1). The main contributors to the study are listed with appreciation in the acknowledgement section.

ACKNOWLEDGEMENTS

The ECE secretariat wishes to express its gratitude to Governments and international organizations which have provided valuable contributions to the present study. Government contributions are included mainly in chapter V (see list of 22 countries in chapter V) and material received from many of the international organizations (listed in table VII.1) has been used throughout the text of other chapters.

Many people, either nominated by their Governments as "focal points" or rapporteurs or representing individual international organizations, have significantly helped with the preparation of this study. The ECE secretariat's thanks go, in particular to N. Saranummi, Technical Research Centre of Finland, Tampere, who has generously made available his extensive experience, as well as his personal efforts and "imagination", without which it would not have been possible to finalize the study. The secretariat would also like to acknowledge the considerable assistance provided by M. Fuchs (United States Department of Commerce) in gathering and selecting unique information, which has proved to be of basic relevancy and value to the present study.

It is a pleasure, also, to offer thanks to the Chairman and Vice-Chairman of both ad hoc Meetings for the study held at Geneva, in 1984 [4] and 1986 [8], N. Richter (Medicor Works, Budapest, current IFMBE president) and R. Kadefors (Projekt Lindholmen, Göteborg), for their excellent conduct of the work and their enthusiasm for the selected subject of digital imaging.

Amongst many individuals who made important comments on the study and/or provided useful information, the following deserve special gratitude (they are listed in alphabetical order, without their titles, positions, etc.):
L. Ambroz (VUZT-CHIRANA, Brno), E. Bengtsson (IMTEC, Uppsala), Y. Bizais (Regional Hospital Centre, Nantes), J.-P. Brotons-Dias (IEC secretariat), J.F. Cornhill (The Ohio State University), I. Eidheim (Directorate of Health, Oslo), L.J. van Erning (St. Radboud Teaching Hospital, Nijmegen), K.-H. Höhne (University Hospital Hamburg-Eppendorf), T.A. Iinuma (National Institute of Radiological Sciences, Chiba-shi), M. Iio (University of Tokyo), P. Jones (ISO secretariat), K. Kita (Toshiba Corporation, Tochigi-ken), H.-U. Lemke (Technical University, Berlin), J. Mallard (University of Aberdeen), D. Meyer-Ebrecht (Technical University, Aachen), R. Millner (Martin-Luther University, Halle-Wittenberg), Laura Lee Murphy (NEMA, Washington), S. Olsson (SPRI, Stockholm), M. Onoe (University of Tokyo), L.F. Pau (Battelle, Geneva), J.F. Place (Battelle, Geneva), S. Rannikko (Centre for Radiation Safety in Finland), R. Renoulin (CCETT, Cesson-Sevigne), M. Saito (University of Tokyo), S. Schuy (Technical University, Graz), N. Slark (DHSS, London), A. Stravs (IFORS/ETH, Zurich), E. Takenaka (National Defense Medical College, Tokorozawa-shi), A. Todd-Pokropek (University College, London), O. Troukhanov (All-Union Medical Engineering Research Institute, Moscow), T. Vadas (Ministry of Industry, Budapest), J.P.J. de Valk (BAZIS/EuroPACS, Leiden), J. Vang (WHO, Regional Office, Copenhagen), P. Vittay (Postgraduate Medical School, Budapest).

The active participation of the above "international team" of experts has been complemented by the work and results of many others, cited in references.

Last but not least, thanks must go to Toshiba Corporation for an idea used in the design of the cover page for the study.

Note: Mention of any manufacturing company or other institution in the context of the present study does not imply endorsement by the United Nations.

LIST OF MAIN ABBREVIATIONS

ACR	American College of Radiology (United States)
BBI	Biomedical Business International
BRS	Basic Radiological System (WHO)
CART	Computer Aided Radiotherapy (Nordic countries)
CCD	Charge couple device
CCETT	Centre commun d'études de télédiffusion et télécommunications (France)
CMEA	Council of Mutual Economic Assistance
CRT	Cathode-ray tube
CSN	Abbreviation for Czechoslovak State standard
CT	Computed tomography
DA	Digital angiography
DBS	Data base system
DBMS	Data base management system
DHSS	Department of Health and Social Security (United Kingdom)
DI	Digital imaging
DIP	Digital image processing
DOR	Digital optical recording
DRG	Diagnosis-related group
DSA	Digital subtraction angiography
DWS	Diagnostic work-station
ECG	Electrocardiography
EEG	Electroencephalography
EFMI	European Federation for Medical Informatics
EFOMP	European Federation of Organizations in Medical Physics
ESR	European Society on Radiology
EuroPACS	European PACS Society (see also PACS)
FDA	Food and Drug Administration (United States)
FDI	International Dental Federation
GNP	Gross national product
GOST	Abbreviation for USSR State standard
HIS	Hospital information system
IAEA	International Atomic Energy Agency
IAMLT	International Association of Medical Laboratory Technologies
IBI	Institute of Biomedical Information
ICRP	International Commission on Radiological Protection
ICRU	International Commission on Radiation Units and Measurements
IDS	Image display station
IEC	International Electrotechnical Commission
IEEE	Institute of Electrical and Electronics Engineers
IFAC	International Federation of Automatic Control
IFIP	International Federation for Information Processing
IFMBE	International Federation for Medical and Biological Engineering
IFORS	International Federation of Operational Research Societies
IIASA	International Institute of Applied Systems Analysis
IIMEBE	International Institute for Medical Electronics and Biological Engineering
IMEKO	International Measurement Confederation
IMIA	International Medical Informatics Association
INICR	International Non-Ionizing Radiation Commission
IOMP	International Organization for Medical Physics
IRPA	International Radiation Protection Association

ISCEV	International Society for Clinical Electrophysiology of Vision
ISFC	International Society and Federation of Cardiology
ISMR	International Society for Magnetic Resonance
ISNM	International Society for Nuclear Medicine
ISO	International Organization for Standardization
ISR	International Society on Radiology
ISTAHC	International Society of Technology Assessment in Health Care
IUPESM	International Union of Physical and Engineering Sciences in Medicine
JAAME	Japan Association for the Advancement of Medical Equipment
LAN	Local area network
MIS	Medical information system
MRI	Magnetic resonance imaging
NEMA	National Electrical Manufacturers Association (United States)
NIH	National Institute of Health (United States)
NMR	Nuclear magnetic resonance
OSI	Open systems interconnections (ISO)
OTA	Office of Technology Assessment (United States)
PACS	Picture archiving and communication system
PET	Positron-emission tomography
QA	Quality assurance
RAM	Random access memory
RIA	Radio-immuno-assay
RIS	Radiological information system
SPECT	Single photon emission computed tomography
SPET	Single photon emission tomography
SPRI	Swedish Planning and Rationalization Institute of Health and Social Services
STU	Swedish National Board for Technical Development
VLSI	Very large-scale integration
VUZT	Research institute of CHIRANA Company (Czechoslovakia)
WFUMB	World Federation of Ultrasound in Medicine and Biology
WHO	World Health Organization

Other symbols employed

*   estimate

.   not applicable

...   not available

-     magnitude zero

1. DEFINITION OF MEDICAL EQUIPMENT

1.1 <u>Health care</u>

Access to adequate health care is comparable to the fundamental rights of human beings. This view has led to the development of large and sophisticated health-care systems. The health-care system comprises primary-care centres and hospitals. Patients enter the system generally through the primary-care centres and are referred to hospitals if they require specialist services for diagnosis and/or therapy. On the primary-care level relatively little medical equipment is used whereas in hospitals it is used extensively.

Health-care expenditures, which account at present for a significant portion (5-11 per cent) of gross national product (GNP), have been increasing over the past decades in many countries at a rate exceeding the growth of overall GNP. Table I.1 provides an example of health care expenditures in one country (United States). The total cost of health care in the United States amounted to over 10 per cent of GNP in 1983, and the estimated growth rate (9.2 per cent) exceeds by far the estimated rate of inflation.

It is generally believed that advances in medical technology are among the major factors fuelling this growth. While the impact of technology continues to be a driving force behind innovation in health-care delivery, factors of equal importance are efforts aimed at making the current technologies less costly and at imposing cost-effectiveness criteria for new technologies. In this respect, public expectations concerning the improved quality of health care should not be underestimated.

Table I.1. United States health-care expenditures, 1983-1988

Type of expenditure	1983 (billions of US dollars)	1985*	1988*	1983-1988 (annual percentage change)
Hospital care	147.2	170.6	228.8	9.2
Physicians' services	69.0	83.9	110.0	9.8
Dentists' services	21.8	27.3	35.2	10.1
Other professional services	8.0	9.8	12.9	10.0
Drugs and medical sundries	23.7	28.1	36.2	8.8
Eyeglasses and appliances	6.2	7.6	9.7	9.3
Nursing-home care	28.8	34.6	46.2	9.9
Other health services	8.5	10.8	14.1	10.7
Programme administration and net cost of insurance	15.6	15.8	19.9	5.0
Government public health activities	11.2	13.8	18.4	10.4
HEALTH SERVICES AND SUPPLIES	340.1	402.4	531.5	9.3
Research	6.2	7.3	8.8	7.3
Construction	9.1	9.9	12.1	5.8
RESEARCH AND CONSTRUCTION OF MEDICAL FACILITIES	15.3	17.2	20.9	6.4
Total public health care personal health care	355.4 313.3	419.5 372.8	552.4 493.3	9.2 9.5

Source: Biomedical Business International, vol. VIII, 1985, p.150.

The national health care systems can be compared, for instance, on the basis of statistics. Table I.2 gives an example of such a comparison. It should be emphasized that these indicators must be complemented by indicators of effectiveness of treatment in order to obtain a balanced picture.

Table I.2: Health-care indicators in selected countries

Indicator	United States	Fed. Rep. of Germany	France	Japan	United Kingdom
Estimated 1984 health expenditure per person (US dollars)	1,500	900	800	500	400
Number of doctors per 100,000 a/	192	222	172	128	154
Life expectancy at birth a/	75	73	76	77	74
Infant mortality per 1,000 live births a/	12	13	10	7	12
Deaths from heart disease per 100,000 a/	435	584	380	266	578

Source: Biomedical Business International, vol. VIII, 1985, p.96. (Original source: The Economist, 1984).

a/ Latest available years.

A more detailed and updated picture of the situation in France, the United Kingdom and the Federal Republic of Germany is given in table I.3.

Table I.3: Selected health-care indicators in
France, the United Kingdom and the
Federal Republic of Germany

Indicator	France	United Kingdom	Federal Republic of Germany
Population (million)	54	56	62
Projected annual population growth, 1980-2000 (percentage)	0.5	0.2	0.1
Health expenditures as percentage of GNP	8.5	5.8	9.4
Health expenditures per capita (US dollars)	853	493	1 000
Doctors per 10,000 inhabitants	21.8	16.1	23.7
Hospital beds per 10,000 inhabitants	111	80	111
Hospital personnel	817 000	782 000	999 000
Occupancy rate of acute beds (percentage)	74.8	71.4	83.0
Average length of stay (days)	9.5	8.3	14.9

Source: Biomedical Business International, vol. VIII, 1985, p. 156.
(Original source: BBI EUROCARE book).

1.2 Diagnosis in medical treatment

The components of health care are:

- Preventive medicine. Averting or protecting persons from the
occurrence of a particular condition or disorder, and forecasting
and/or identifying the individuals at risk of acquiring a particular
illness at some time in the future;

- Diagnosis. Determining the nature and circumstances of a disease
condition through examination, tests, evaluation of information and
monitoring;

- Therapy. Deciding on how to treat the patient for the diagnosed
disease condition with a combination of curative, supportive and/or
interventional processes, and the treatment; and

- Rehabilitation. Restoring or re-establishing a condition of good
health, the ability to work, or integration into society, ideally at
the level that existed before the illness.

The critical element in this chain is diagnosis. Once a physician makes a diagnosis and institutes therapy, diagnostic procedures are used to monitor therapy and assess the adequacy of response to measures designed to optimize rehabilitation and prevention.

Diagnostic capabilities directly affect the design and definition of preventive measures and therapies. For example, it is quite likely that diseases such as toxic shock syndrome, acquired immune deficiency syndrome, adult respiratory stress syndrome and others have been in existence for some time, but the ability to identify and detect them did not exist until recently.

Early disease detection usually affords more satisfactory results in terms of disease outcome and recovery. Despite significant advances, there are still numerous problems in diagnostic technology. For example, diagnosis is a sequential process, with each step focusing more closely on the nature of the illness. However, diagnostic tests have a limited sensitivity and specificity and therefore diagnostic precision requires various complementing tests. Economic practicalities limit the spectrum of tests available. Finally, the complexity of data resulting from a series of tests may prove difficult for the physician to interpret.

Thus, automated processes that rapidly, non-invasively and inexpensively generate physiological and/or anatomical data are preferred. The stage is set for advances that provide new and more precise data more easily and more cheaply than by present methods. At the same time, great caution should be applied in advocating mass-screening procedures in view of the risk of obtaining imprecise medical data, as mentioned above.

1.3 Biomedical equipment markets

Table I.4 summarizes the market situation for health-care products in some parts of the world in 1983 (estimated values).

Table I.4: **Health-care markets in the United States, Japan and some**
European countries in 1983 (estimated values) (including
all devices, diagnostics, equipment and supplies and
excluding services)

Country	Population (millions)	Health-care expenditures			
		US dollars per capita	Products (million US dollars)	Imported (percentage)	Growth rate (percentage) a/
United States	236	1,500	14,500	20	6-8
Japan	120	500	3,050	20	2-3
Fed. Rep. of Germany	62	950	1,750	55	4-5
France	55	800	1,050	60	4-5
United Kingdom	56	450	950	40	2-3
Italy	58	340	800	45	2-3
Spain	39	300	300	60	2-3
Other selected	80	400	1,600	60	4-5
Total	706	858	24,000	.	.

Source: *Biomedical Business International*, vol. VII, 1984, p.192.

a/ Estimated average annual rate of growth for medical product imports 1983-1987.

Extrapolating from that, the total world market is shared geographically approximately as follows: United States: 50 per cent; Japan: 10 per cent; western Europe: 25 per cent; and other: 15 per cent.

Table I.5 shows the distribution of shipments between various equipment categories in the United States.

Value of shipments of medical and dental instruments in the United States, 1983-1986

(Millions of US dollars)

SIC group	1983	1984 a/	1985 b/	1986 c/
X-ray apparatus and tubes	4 565	4 661	4 926	5 621
Surgical and medical instruments	4 343	4 495	4 617	4 857
Surgical appliances and supplies	6 044	6 473	6 615	6 847
Dental equipment and supplies	1 117	1 147	1 178	1 213
Total shipments	16 069	16 776	17 336	18 538

Source: 1986 U.S. Industrial Outlook; U.S. Department of Commerce, International Trade Administration (ITA), Washington 1986.

a/ Estimates except for exports and imports.

b/ Estimates.

c/ Forecast.

Table I.6 illustrates the geographic structure of United States international trade in the field of medical and dental instruments.

Table I.6. Top United States trading partners in medical and dental instruments in 1984 (five leaders for each category)

(Percentage of total)

Country	X-ray and electromedical equipment		Surgical and medical instruments		Surgical appliances and supplies		Dental equipment and supplies		Total medical and dental instruments	
	Exports	Imports	Exports	Imports	Exports	Imports	Exports	Imports	Exports	Imports
Canada	12	...	18	...	19	8	21	7	16	...
Denmark	...	...	...	...	...	10	...	...	...	...
Germany, Fed. Rep. of	11	32	6	19	8	25	10	28	9	28
Ireland	...	...	...	...	...	...	...	5	...	...
Israel	...	10	...	...	...	...	...	...	...	6
Italy	...	...	...	...	...	...	6	...	...	...
Japan	13	20	10	37	9	8	11	28	11	23
Mexico	...	...	...	8	...	8	...	...	...	...
Netherlands	8	8	7	...	7	...	...	...	7	5
Saudi Arabia	...	...	7	...	...	...	...	...	...	...
Singapore	...	...	...	9	...	...	...	...	...	...
Switzerland	...	...	...	...	...	11	5	11	...	...
United Kingdom	9	7	8	5	10	...	...	...	9	6

Source: 1986 U.S. Industrial Outlook; U.S. Department of Commerce, International Trade Administration (ITA), Washington 1986.

More detailed figures on production and trade in electromedical and radiation equipment, including X-ray, in the United States are presented in chapter V.

1.4 Types of medical equipment

The spectrum of medical equipment is broad. Generally it is categorized into diagnostic and therapeutic equipment and broken down into the following subgroups:-

- Diagnostic

    - Bioelectric recording equipment (e.g. ECG and EEG)

    - Monitoring equipment (e.g. for ECG, blood pressure and circulation)

    - Endoscopic equipment

    - Laboratory equipment for the analysis of patient samples (e.g. in clinical chemistry, haematology, microbiology and pathology)

    - Imaging equipment (e.g. X-ray and ultrasound)

- Therapeutic

    - Anaesthesia equipment (e.g. respirators)

    - Surgical equipment (e.g. surgical diathermy)

    - Physiatric equipment (e.g. therapeutic ultrasound)

    - Radiation therapy (e.g. linear accelerators)

    - Devices implanted under the skin or worn by the patient (e.g. artificial organs, pacemakers and insulin infusion pumps)

    - Other therapeutic equipment (e.g. haemodialysis equipment, defibrillators and infusion pumps)

However, this breakdown is incomplete, overlapping and artificial. The grouping is made more difficult by the emergence of new systems combining various techniques, e.g. an endoscope combined with a surgical diathermy unit. Another division breaks down medical equipment into patient-connected and non-patient-connected equipment. This division is used in connection with safety standards for electromedical equipment. A non-exhaustive list of equipment categorized as electromedical equipment is provided in the annex of IEC Publication 601-1. [10]

In the past decade, the emphasis in medical equipment has shifted from the application of microelectronics to system-level solutions. This includes the incorporation of computers and associated software in existing products and the integration of these systems through local area networks (LAN) and software into medical information systems (MIS). Attempts to integrate the existing isolated departmental medical information systems into a hospital information system (HIS) have underlined the importance of top-down planning. This problem is no different from the one experienced in other application areas, like office or factory automation.

Apart from information technology, material sciences are also having a major impact on medical equipment and devices. This is particularly noted in the case of artificial organs. New ceramic and polymer materials are better accepted by the body, and are more reliable and lighter.

Roughly, imaging and laboratory equipment make up approximately 30 and 40 per cent, respectively, of the total value of medical equipment in a hospital. The remaining 30 per cent is shared between the other device groups.

2. GENERAL TRENDS IN ADVANCED MEDICAL EQUIPMENT AND SYSTEMS

2.1 Health care and cost-effectiveness analysis

The organizational structure of health care comprises, in descending order, policy-makers, health administrators, clinical decision-makers (diagnosis and therapy), operative personnel to carry out the decisions and technical staff for the support of the technologies used. This last group contains the so-called clinical engineers and hospital physicists that provide advice, help and service in the effective utilization of complex medical devices.

In recent years, health-care expenditure has tended to rise annually by more than the inflation rate and has in many countries reached a level where additional increases are not so readily accepted. As a consequence of this, the following questions are surfacing with increasing frequency: What is good health? What is good-quality health care? What is cost-effective health care? What can we (individuals, local and State governments, firms) afford to pay, given other demands on resources?

Reflecting this concern over increasing costs, various cost-containment schemes have been developed in a number of countries. In the United States, the Federal Government has introduced into the Medicare programme diagnosis-related groups (DRG) making diagnosis the key factor in reimbursement. Under the DRG system, the provider receives the same fee (regardless of services performed) for each patient with the same diagnosis. This gives providers an incentive to deliver as few services as possible in order to minimize costs. Liability considerations and accepted medical standards ensure that optimal diagnostic capability is made available.

Following the example of the United States, several other countries with similar health-care systems are planning to introduce DRGs.

The Regional Office for Europe of the World Health Organization (WHO) has for several years been advocating the appropriate use of medical technology. Recently it organized a meeting on Budgetary Incentives for the Appropriate Use of Medical Technology, (Cologne, Federal Republic of Germany, 8 to 11 October 1984). The meeting provided a forum where representatives of several countries reported on national efforts and experiences in meeting the requirement for rationalization of health-care services. The conclusion was reached that physician behaviour related to the appropriate use of medical technology could be substantially modified.

The innovations in the beginning of the 1970s leading to the first commercial computed tomography (CT) scanner and the subsequent rapid diffusion of this technology into clinical practice highlighted the problem of establishing criteria for the appropriate use of certain technologies in health care. [11] A new interdisciplinary field of science incorporating health economics, medical, sociological and technical sciences has resulted from that concern, namely technology assessment in health care. Assessments of CT technology were carried out in the late 1970s by the Office of Technology Assessment (OTA) of the United States Congress [12] and by the Planning and Rationalization Institute for Health Care (SPRI, Sweden). [13] Subsequently this activity was taken over by many others and now plays an important part in the introduction of new medical technologies. In many countries, consensus development seminars on various medical technologies (e.g. use of diagnostic ultrasound during pregnancy, hip-joint replacement and coronary by-pass surgery) have been organized. Early in 1985, an International Society for Technology Assessment in Health Care (ISTAHC) was established with its own journal. [14]

Technology assessments are intended to provide information for policy-makers and health administrators of the appropriate level of diffusion of selected technologies (both adoption and utilization) in health care. Quality assurance of the care provided to patients (both diagnostic and therapeutic services) has been a topic of international co-operation between physicians since the beginning of this century, when the international society was established.

An important thing to remember in considering health-care costs is that most of them are incurred by elderly people. In fact, 50 per cent of the average consumer's lifetime expenditures on health care occur during the last year of the consumer's life. In all countries, the group of elderly persons will expand considerably compared with the other age groups during the next 20 to 30 years. This will increase the demands for health care and make it even more important to evaluate and redirect present methods and technologies for health care.

One indication of this is the emphasis put on home-health-care techniques in many countries. Technologies that enable individuals to continue living independently at home are being encouraged. The problem of the elderly is connected to that of the handicapped. Technically speaking, both groups are handicapped and need technical aids for independent living, or as someone has said "tools for living". [15] The amount and the degree of sophistication of these technologies varies in accordance with the degree of handicap that needs to be compensated.

2.2 Advanced medical equipment and systems

Science and technology are evolving rapidly. This creates the potential for applying these innovations also to health-care products. Improved and/or cheaper older technologies and products, and sometimes even new ones, will continue to emerge as a consequence of this. On the basis of medical, economic and technical assessments, the users should decide which old technologies should be replaced and which new ones put into use.

The concept of "advanced" in this context is understood to refer to innovative products. They can be technologically complicated or simple. Examples of these include:

- Artificial organs, such as heart valves, hip-joints and implanted pacemakers. In this area, material sciences, reliability and durability are key factors;

- Patient-monitoring equipment, comprising sophisticated transducers, such as transcutaneous oxygen transducers, together with microelectronics, microprocessors and software for processing the measured signals;

- Information systems for patient-data management and for decision support integrating various sources of patient data and incorporating, for example, knowledge-based techniques (artificial intelligence, expert systems) for the interpretation of the compiled data. Such systems are used and developed for intensive care, clinical laboratories, etc.;

- Imaging of the anatomy and functions of the human body, a rapidly expanding area where many imaging modalities are currently available. The technology for obtaining and storing the images is changing from film to digital. Integration of the various image sources with picture archiving and communicating systems (PACS) and image processing stations is the present trend;

- Automated laboratory equipment for the processing of patient samples (blood, urine, etc.), an area that has been highly cost-effective. It incorporates many technologies necessary in the handling, dispensing, incubation and analysis of the samples. Information systems are extensively used to manage the process, for quality control and for producing laboratory reports to wards and treating physicians. The ease with which these analyses can be performed led at one point to undue proliferation of this technology; and

- Technical aids for the handicapped (and for the elderly), comprising both simple and complex tools. Lately, developments in information technology and in robotics have opened up new possibilities in environmental control and communication both at home and at work.

2.3 Organizational and operational aspects in connection with advanced medical equipment

The introduction of high-technology medical equipment into health care requires changes to be made in the training of the staff and in the ways of operation, in order to utilize and maintain the equipment efficiently.

High-technology equipment normally requires more skills from the user although at the same time it relieves him of trivial routine tasks. To control the correct functioning of the system, one has to understand its basic operation principles and be able to apply some quality (performance) assurance tests for that purpose. The physicians utilizing the results produced with this equipment need to understand the limitations of the technology, e.g. as concerns its sensitivity and specificity. Both basic and on-site training need to be adapted to accommodate these additional requirements. The efficient use of a technology also requires motivation from the users. An important step towards achieving this is adequate training.

It must be noted that hands-on training in the use of specific equipment is generally very much neglected in health care, although international standards stress the importance of instructions for use. [16]

The effective utilization of high-technology equipment and systems necessitates the technical expertise of clinical engineers, hospital physicists and/or computer scientists.

The efficient and cost-effective utilization of a new technology also requires careful planning in organization and ways of operation. This includes consideration of what are the appropriate hierarchical levels in health-care for a new technology, and whether it should be centralized or decentralized. A good example of a decentralized technology is ultrasonic imaging, which is widely used in obstetrics, cardiology and radiology.

High-technology equipment requires regular servicing, one reason being that it usually incorporates computer equipment. Many studies have shown that regular preventive maintenance combined with performance assurance procedures is more cost-effective than reliance on repair. [17] This servicing can be done either by an institution hiring its own personnel or by an outside contractor.

The installation of new equipment or technology can be expensive in terms of both additional staff requirements and actual purchasing and installation costs, e.g. installation of a magnetic resonance imaging (MRI) system may be especially costly, depending on the type of magnet used, whereas ultrasonic imagers have no installation costs.

2.4 Justification for selecting digital imaging as a subject area for the study

The criteria for selecting DI as the subject area can be analysed from a clinical and an industrial point of view. Within medical engineering, DI is a good example of a highly interdisciplinary and high-technology area that is experiencing fast development. In recent years, new imaging modalities have emerged, such as magnetic resonance imaging (MRI), positron emission tomography (PET), ultrasonic imaging and digital angiography (DA). While the old techniques such as conventional X-ray, computed tomography (CT) and nuclear imaging with gamma cameras still exist, the new techniques are clinically superior in diagnosing certain diseases and require a shorter stay in hospital.

Besides diagnostic imaging, DI has potential in many other medical fields, such as cell and chromosome analysis in microscopy, photo- and densitometry and visualization of multi-dimensional signals and features.

Developments in information technology are applied to diagnostic imaging as well. All imaging devices except the conventional film-based X-ray produce digital images. This will result in the integration of image sources through local area networks, picture archives and image processing stations (in short, PACS).

The new diagnostic imaging modalities are all costly as far as purchase, installation, use and maintenance are concerned. To achieve cost-effectiveness, careful planning and evaluation are necessary.

The health-care viewpoint may be summarized in the following questions:

(i)   What is the economic equation (cost-effectiveness)?

(ii) In which cases should each imaging modality be used? and

(iii) What is the optimum diffusion of each technology?

For industry, the problems can be divided into two categories:
technological and commercial. The technologies are evolving rapidly,
resulting in shorter product lives. The development of new products requires
much capital, know-how, the mastering of several technologies
(microelectronics, physics, computers, pattern recognition, control theory,
software development, etc.) and close co-operation with users and research.
Since the field is evolving and expanding rapidly, internationally-recognized
standards for interfacing equipment with other systems are only just emerging.

On the other hand, the market potential of DI is very high for new
imaging modalities and image handling. However, uncertainty prevails
concerning the willingness of the health-care system to pay for these
expansions.

CHAPTER II - DEFINITION AND STATE OF THE ART OF DIGITAL IMAGE GENERATION AND PROCESSING EQUIPMENT AND SYSTEMS

1. CHARACTERISTICS OF DIGITAL IMAGING EQUIPMENT AND SYSTEMS - SPECTRUM

Wilhelm C. Röntgen discovered electromagnetic radiation in 1895. X-rays have been in use in medical diagnosis since the beginning of the century. With the advent of digital imaging (DI), however, the field has developed and diversified considerably, especially within the past 20 years. Figure II.1. illustrates the present situation from the DI viewpoint, and the integration of DI devices through the picture archiving and communication system (PACS). The range of devices able to produce digital diagnostic images is broad, as shown in the figure. At present the connection of these imaging devices through a PACS is not readily possible as standardized interfaces and protocols are only just coming into use (e.g. the ACR-NEMA standard). The resolution of the images (number of pixels, pixel resolution, etc.) also varies.

Digital imaging devices can be divided into image sources and image sinks (table II.1). Some modules can act both as sources and as sinks, for example, the image archive and the diagnostic image processing station.

A PACS can be connected to other PACS, as in figure II.1, where it is connected to the PACS of the radiotherapy clinic. Referring physicians have access to images and reports through image-display stations that do not have all the image-handling possibilities of the diagnostic work-stations (DWS) used by the specialist physicians (e.g. radiologists). The variety of image work-stations needed on clinical practice will be established through clinical testing and evaluation of research concepts.

Figure II.1 omits one important imaging device: the conventional film-based X-ray, since it is not digital. It can be interfaced with the DI system via the film digitizer/densitometer. The multiformat camera of table II.1 is used to store digital images on film.

Apart from diagnostic imaging as presented in figure II.1, DI in medicine has found applications in the microscopic analysis of cells. These include automation of the differential count in haematology, classification of tissue samples in pathology, etc. In these applications, the main emphasis has been on pattern recognition, whereas in digital diagnostic imaging the acquisition of images has so far been the main problem area.

Other medical applications include image processing in connection with radiotherapy, where the localization of the tumour, treatment planning for its irradiation and subsequent simulation and check and confirm operations all involve DI techniques.

Digital imaging can also be useful in surgical operations such as neurosurgery. The final outcome in this area could be a surgical robot with a vision system making possible high-precision surgical operations. [18] Visualization of phenomena measured - e.g. as time-varying signals - is also an interesting application. The localization and spreading of brain activity caused by external stimuli can be visualized using electroencephalogram or magnetoencephalogram recordings.

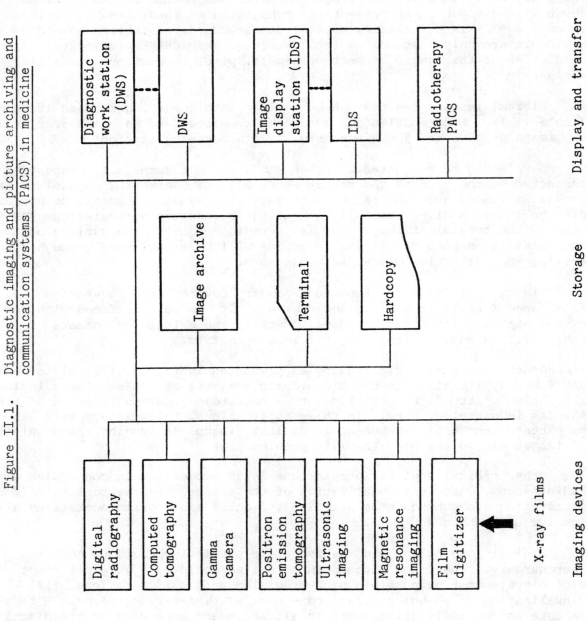

Figure II.1. Diagnostic imaging and picture archiving and communication systems (PACS) in medicine

- 24 -

Table II.1. Classification of digital imaging devices into those that produce images (sources) and those that use them (sinks)

Device	Image source	Image sink	Image source/sink	Neither
Digital radiography unit	X			
Computed tomography	X		X	
Digital subtraction angiographic system	X		X	
Gamma camera	X		X	
Ultrasound systems	X			
Magnetic resonance imaging	X		X	
Positron-emission tomography	X		X	
Film digitizer/densitometer	X			
Multiformat camera		X		
Diagnostic work-station		X	X	
Image archive			X	
Image-display station		X		
Printer (hard copy)		X		
Management terminal				X
Connection to other PACS	X	X	X	

Source: ACR-NEMA Digital Imaging and Communications Standard.

Outside the field of medicine, the applications of DI are also numerous. They include the use of satellite-mounted imaging systems for land resource analysis and planning, weather forecasts and military purposes; image transfer systems to transmit images over long distances; security systems for the identification of signatures, fingerprints or faces; robotics and industrial process control with intelligent vision systems. An in-depth discussion of these is outside the scope of this study. These applications serve to increase the rate of development of DI technologies since they make the whole field of DI more attractive to industry and help the development of image analysis and compression and transmission methods on a broad scale. Figure II.2 illustrates the structure and characteristics of image technologies in general.

Owing to the latest developments in microcomputer-based image processing boards and larger software compatibility, DI industrial and scientific applications have found wide diffusion in various areas such as:

- Enhancing the grey-scale detail in images produced by various medical imaging devices;

- Recognizing patterns for real-time inspection of industrial parts and products as well as for some other manufacturing operations;

- Comparing several digitized images, or different aspects of the same image, with a reference image;

Figure II.2. Image technology characteristics

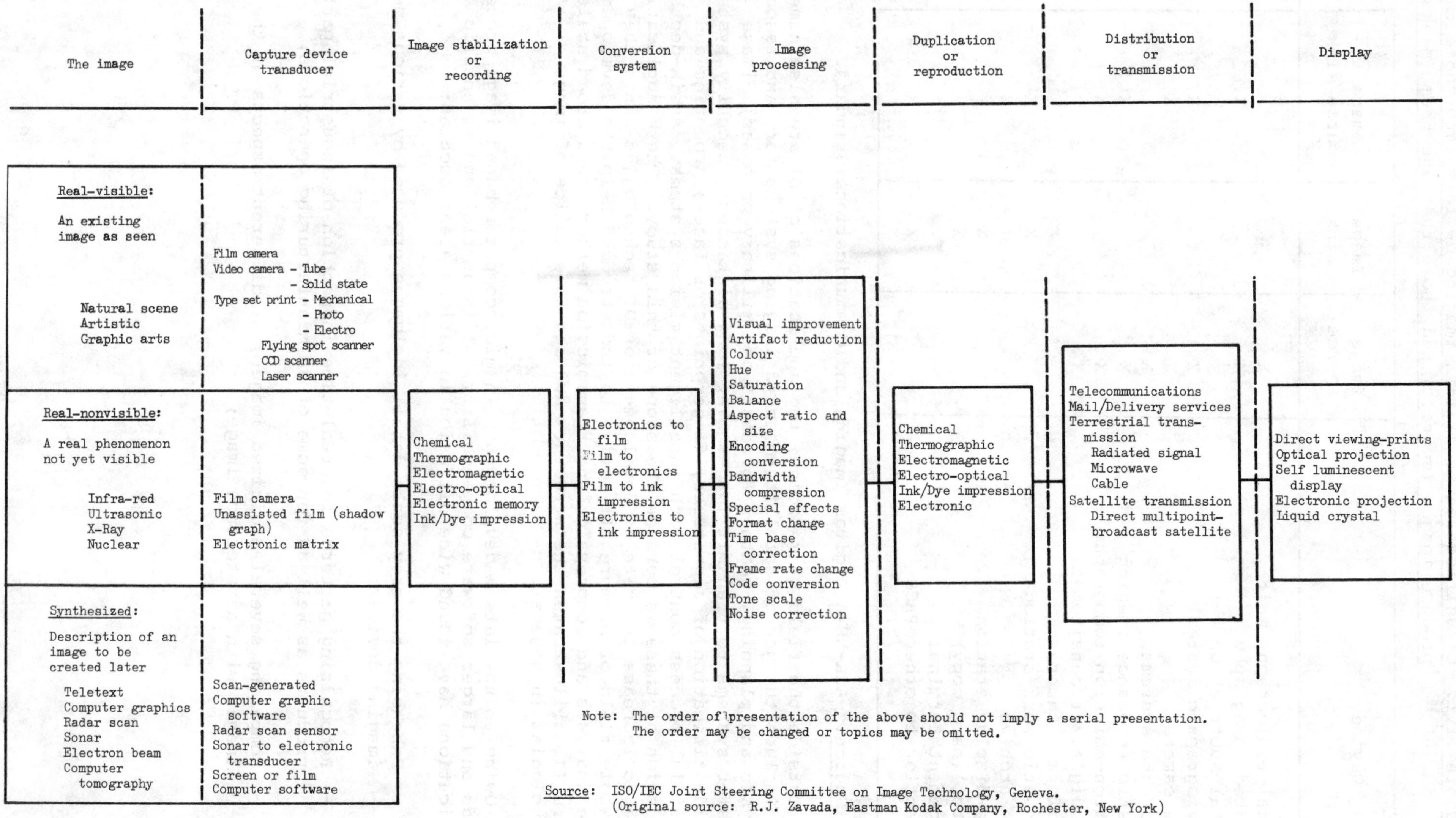

The image	Capture device transducer	Image stabilization or recording	Conversion system	Image processing	Duplication or reproduction	Distribution or transmission	Display
Real-visible: An existing image as seen Film camera Video camera – Tube – Solid state Type set print – Mechanical – Photo – Electro Flying spot scanner CCD scanner Laser scanner Natural scene Artistic Graphic arts		Chemical Thermographic Electromagnetic Electro-optical Electronic memory Ink/Dye impression	Electronics to film Film to electronics Film to ink impression Electronics to ink impression	Visual improvement Artifact reduction Colour Hue Saturation Balance Aspect ratio and size Encoding conversion Bandwidth compression Special effects Format change Time base correction Frame rate change Code conversion Tone scale Noise correction	Chemical Thermographic Electromagnetic Electro-optical Ink/Dye impression Electronic	Telecommunications Mail/delivery services Terrestrial transmission Radiated signal Microwave Cable Satellite transmission Direct multipoint-broadcast satellite	Direct viewing-prints Optical projection Self luminescent display Electronic projection Liquid crystal
Real-nonvisible: A real phenomenon not yet visible Infra-red Ultrasonic X-Ray Nuclear	Film camera Unassisted film (shadow graph) Electronic matrix						
Synthesized: Description of an image to be created later Teletext Computer graphics Radar scan Sonar Electron beam Computer tomography	Scan-generated Computer graphic software Radar scan sensor Sonar to electronic transducer Screen or film Computer software						

Note: The order of presentation of the above should not imply a serial presentation. The order may be changed or topics may be omitted.

Source: ISO/IEC Joint Steering Committee on Image Technology, Geneva. (Original source: R.J. Zavada, Eastman Kodak Company, Rochester, New York)

- Detecting motion for industrial control and security applications; and

- Transmitting images in-house or to remote sites for
  teleconferencing. [19]

Since the main applications of DI in medicine are in diagnostic imaging, this area will be the focus of the present study. The other applications will be discussed only briefly.

2. X-RAY TECHNOLOGIES

2.1 Film-based X-ray

Conventional X-ray examination techniques still dominate the field of diagnostic imaging, although most of the imagers at present being purchased are digital. The major problem in using ionizing radiation is the radiation dose produced, and in the development of new X-ray techniques the minimization of the radiation dose is one of the goals. The state of the art in the utilization of ionizing radiation for diagnostic and therapeutic purposes (mostly cancer treatment) is illustrated in figure II.3.

Operating principle

X-rays are absorbed by the body in relation to the specific density and atomic number of various tissues. In irradiating a volume of interest, these absorption differences are recorded on film. To decrease the required radiation dose, amplifying plates are used. Some years ago, lantanide-based plates made possible a further reduction of dose. Film development requires personnel and equipment. Malfunctions and faults in development equipment are not uncommon and necessitate frequent quality-assurance checks to sustain an adequate and constant image quality. Technically (resolution and dynamic range) X-ray films are an excellent medium for storing images. However, because they contain silver they are costly and, especially, the film archives are expensive, since in many countries X-ray films are required to be archived for as long as five to ten years.

An alternative to direct film storage is fluoroscopy, where an image intensifier is used to convert the transmitted X-rays into a visible image that can be viewed at the output screen of the image intensifier. By use of a spot camera, the image can then be stored on film. The film is of much smaller size than that used in normal X-ray examinations (100 x 100 mm compared with 400 x 400 mm).

Instead of a spot camera, a cine or video camera can be used, thus making possible the imaging of dynamic phenomena. One such examination is called angiography: the imaging of blood vessels. Angiographic examinations, as well as some others, require the injection of contrast medium into the bloodstream to make the blood vessels visible.

The World Health Organization has strongly encouraged manufacturers to produce an inexpensive and easy-to-use X-ray system (basic radiology system, BRS) for use in developing countries. [20] The system utilizes the latest technology, such as intermediate frequencies to reduce the size of the transformer and the ripple in high voltage. Although primarily intended for developing countries, it could be used in primary care in the developed countries as well.

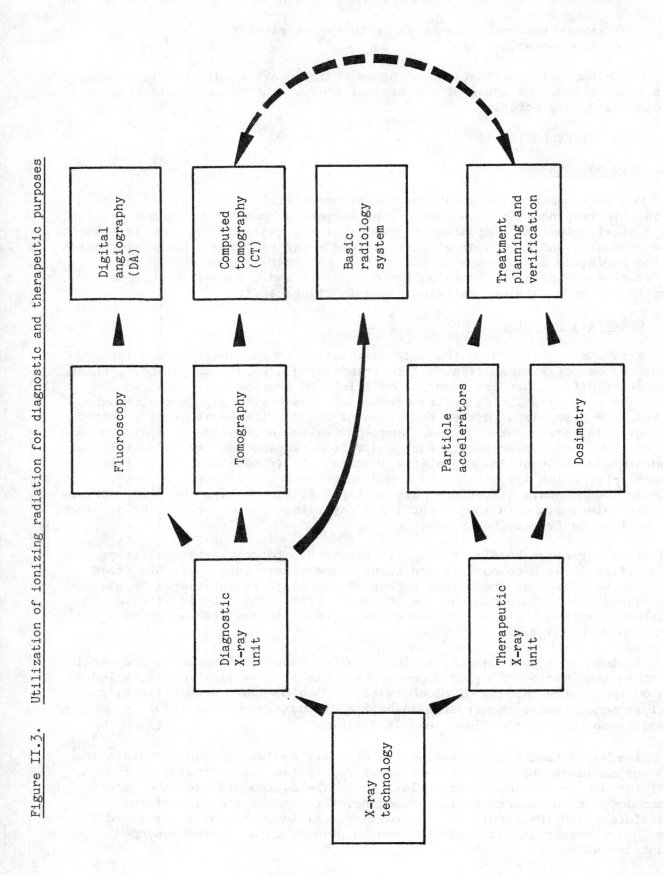

Figure II.3. Utilization of ionizing radiation for diagnostic and therapeutic purposes

Treatment planning procedures of today rely on CT-images.

2.2 Digital radiography

Image-plate technique

In digital radiography the image is recorded in digital form. This can
at present be done either by using the image-plate technique developed by Fuji
or by digitizing the video image obtained in fluoroscopy. In Fuji's computed
radiography technique, an image plate [21] replaces the X-ray film. During
exposure, the image is stored on the plate and can be read with a scanning
monochromatic laser beam (figure II.4). The images can be digitized during
the scanning operation.

The image-plate technique reduces the radiation dose to a tenth or less
of that used with plain films, an important advantage in paediatrics. At
present, both Toshiba and Philips (developing its own system) market the Fuji
image-plate system.

New fully digital techniques

Many researchers are exploring other means of replacing film/screen X-ray
image recording with electronic image detectors in order to reduce scatter
radiation and for economic reasons. Many of these are based on scanning to
obtain a two-dimensional image. The systems are based, for example, on the
flying spot scanner and electronic slit scanners. For the time being these
systems are not commercially available.

Production prototypes of such systems are at present being tested in some
hospitals in the United States. The system comprises e.g. 8,000 detectors
(1,000/inch) and is capable of a resolution of 4,096 x 4,096 pixels with a
dynamic range of 1,024 grey levels. This corresponds to 8 to 10 linepairs
per millimetre.

Digital angiography

Operating principle

In digital angiography (DA) - sometimes called digital subtraction
angiography (DSA) - the image is digitized from the video image. Digital
angiography is a new, rapidly developing technology for diagnosing conditions
associated with the internal structure of blood vessels. It involves
injecting contrast medium into the artery and measuring over time the changing
concentration of contrast medium passing through the vascular structures of
interest. Using a computer, the images before the contrast injection are
subtracted from those after injection to give a numerical representation of
the arterial structure being studied. This technique can be performed with a
very low risk of morbidity compared with conventional and invasive techniques
such as arteriography. Figure II.5 gives the basic block diagram of a
DA system.

Clinical use

Digital angiography has been shown to have important clinical uses in
diagnosing diseases of the carotid, renal, intracranial and peripheral
arteries, the aorta, and pulmonary circulation. It is reasonable to expect
that it will develop to the point where it will have wide applicability in

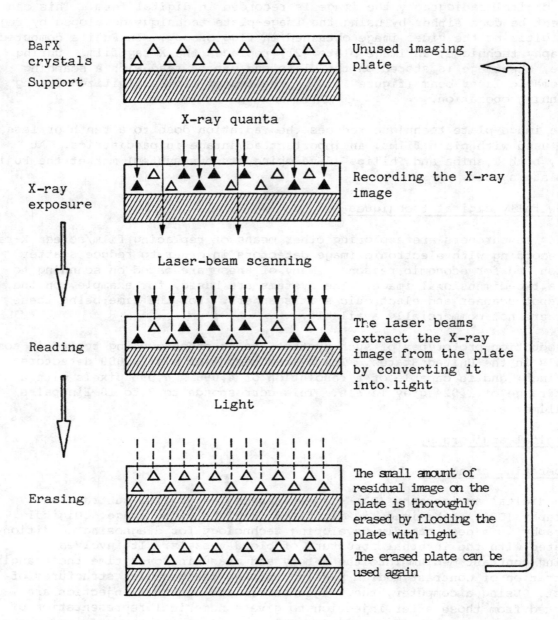

Source: Fuji Photo Film Co. Ltd., Japan.

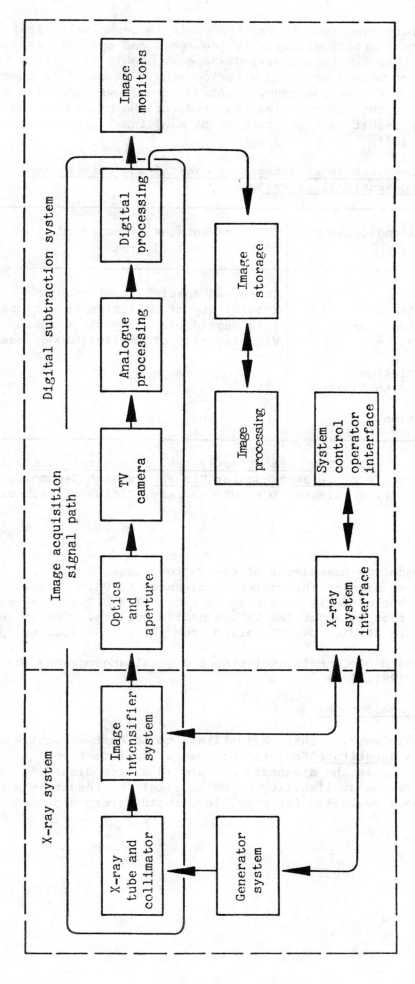

Figure II.5. Diagram of a digital angiography system

Source: M. Menken et al. The Cost Effectiveness of Digital Subtraction Angiography in the Diagnosis of Cerebrovascular Disease (Health Technology Case Study 3V, OTA-HCS-34), Washington D.C: US Congress, Office of Technology Assessment, May 1985.

- 31 -

diagnosing coronary artery disease. At the moment it is technically less
accurate than conventional arteriography. As the speed and spatial resolution
of DA images improves, this limitation will disappear. Table II.2 lists the
comparative advantages of DA and standard arteriography. It is clear that DA
is not yet a substitute for arteriography. Instead, the lower radiation and
complication rates of DA, the reduced time required for the procedure, and
patient acceptance, may result in a use rate of DA many times greater than
that of arteriography. [22]

Table II.2. Comparative advantages of digital angiography and
conventional arteriography

Advantages of digital angiography	Advantages of standard arteriography
Decreased morbidity Decreased patient discomfort Decreased hospitalization time Decreased procedure time Decreased film cost Increased contrast resolution Usefulness in patients with limited arterial access Lower cost per examination	Increased spatial resolution Feasibility of selective injections Less degradation of patient motion Visualization of smaller blood vessels

Source: M. Menken et al. The Cost Effectiveness of Digital Subtraction
Angiography in the Diagnosis of Cerebrovascular Disease (Health Technology
Case Study 3V, OTA-HCS-34), Washington DC: US Congress, Office of Technology
Assessment, May 1985.

Cost-effectiveness

The Office of Technology Assessment of the United States (OTA) has
examined the published studies on the cost-effectiveness of DA. A summary of
these as concerns the cost of DA is presented in table II.3. The break-even
cost without physician fees is about 280 United States dollars. The billed
charges in the literature studied by OTA varied from 175 to 300 dollars.

Another valuable techno-economic analysis of digital angiography was
published in Sweden in 1985. [23]

Future of digital angiography

The OTA study concludes "... that DA is likely to be cost-effective if
its pattern of use is a substitute for, rather than a supplement to,
conventional arteriography in the diagnosis of carotid artery disease". It
also concludes that "... the availability of DA is likely to result in a much
larger number of patients evaluated for possible carotid artery disease". [22]

Table II.3. Costs of digital angiography (physician fees not included)
(US dollars)

Purchase price	
New system (equipment and room) or	4 800 000
Addition to existing fluoroscope equipment	250 000
Utilization costs	
Personnel (2 technicians per case; 2 000 annually)	50 000
Miscellaneous costs	
(administration, insurance, secretaries)	50 000
Supply costs/per case 80 dollars x 2 000 cases	160 000
Break-even cost for 2,000 DAs annually	280

Source: As for table II.2.

2.3 Computed tomography

Operating principle

The computed tomography system (CT scanner) has undergone dramatic changes since the first commercial head scanner was developed in the early 1970s. In computed tomography, a tomographic slice image is reconstructed by a computer algorithm from the absorption values of X-ray radiation when the target is irradiated from various angles. The inventors of the CT technology (G. Hounsfield and A. Cormack) received the Nobel prize in physiology and medicine in 1979. The first scanners required a long scanning time (several minutes) and could be used only to image the head where there was no patient movement. Later, as the technology advanced, scanning times were reduced to a level allowing imaging of the whole body. Table II.4 lists the operating principles and technical specifications according to the motion of the gantry. The improvements characterizing the development of four generations of CT scanners (the fifth-generation cine-scanner is at present being introduced) are illustrated in figures II.6 to II.9.

Improvements in the technology have allowed shorter scan times and increased resolution (some 0.5 mm), minimizing problems associated with patient motion. The spatial resolution of a CT image is still, however, of much lower quality than that of an X-ray film. The dynamic range of a CT image is larger than that of conventional film-based X-ray. Thanks to computer processing, the user can view the image with a self-adjustable dynamic range (either grey or colour scale). In technical terms, the range varies between 8 and 16 bits (256-65,000 grey levels). The image size is normally 512 x 512 pixels (pixel = number of picture elements in an image). The images are stored on magnetic tapes or diskettes. A multiformat camera is used to convert the CRT image on to X-ray film, thus allowing conventional archiving. The improvement achieved in scan speed and in spatial resolution during the last decade is illustrated in figures II.10 and II.11.

Figure II.6. First generation CT
(Pencil beam scanner)

Figure II.7. Second generation CT
(Rectilinear multiple pencil
beam scanner with multiple
degree increments)

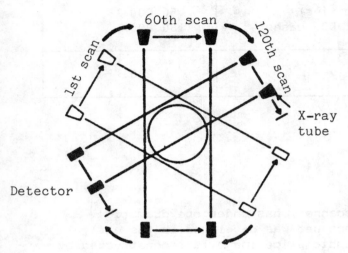

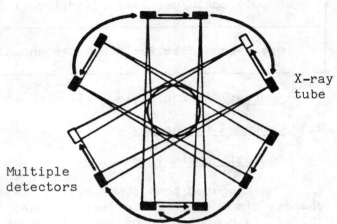

Figure II.8. Third generation CT

Figure II.9. Fourth generation CT

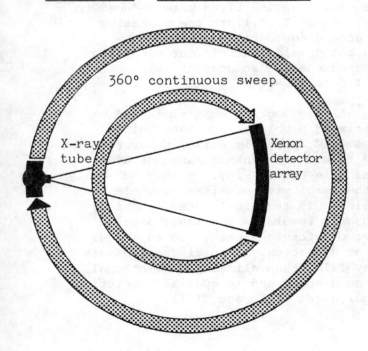

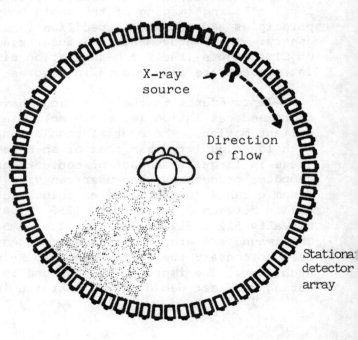

Source for figures II.6-II.9: Diagnostic Imaging, 1986.

Figure II.10. CT scanner - improvement of
scan speed (1975-1985)

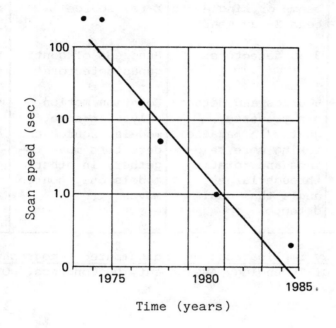

Figure II.11. CT scanner - improvement of
spatial resolution (1975-1985)

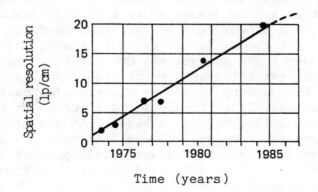

Source for figures II.10-II.11: Diagnostic Imaging, 1986.

- 35 -

Table II.4. Scanner types according to motion of gantry

Rotate and translate, dual detector	Rotate and translate, multiple detector	Rotate only	Electronic rotation
4-6 min scan time	20 s-2 min scan time	Under 5 s scan time	20 ms scan time
Single pencil beam X-ray source	2 or more pencil beams or single fan beam X-ray source	Single fan beam X-ray source	Several fan beam X-ray sources
2 detectors	3-60 detectors	Hundreds of contiguous detectors	Hundreds of contiguous detectors
Source and detectors traverse gantry in parallel, gantry rotates through small angle, process repeats	Sources and detectors traverse gantry in parallel taking more readings and rotating through larger angle than dual detector	Rotation motion only. In some models, source and detectors move together, in other models only source moves	No moving parts. Scan accomplished electronically

Source: Policy implications of the computed tomography (CT) scanner. An updating. Office of Technology Assessment, US Congress. OTA-BP-H-8, January 1981, p.61.

Clinical use

The CT scanner undoubtedly remains a remarkable advance in diagnostic medicine. Following its introduction, it diffused into clinical use very rapidly. In fact, the diffusion was so rapid that health-care providers became worried about the costs and the appropriate level of availability. This led to the development and formal acceptance of technology assessments in medicine. The first assessment reports dealt with CT scanners. [24, 25] The Office of Technology Assessment renewed its study on CT in 1981 concluding, among other things, that the diffusion of CT in the United States was levelling off at around 1,500 operational CT scanners. [26] However, more recent data indicates that this was not the case. In 1983 there were approximately 6,000 CT scanners in use on a world-wide basis, of which 2,400 were in the United States. [27] Figure II.12 illustrates the diffusion of CT in Sweden, where no levelling off is in sight. At the time of the OTA study, the number of CT scanners in Sweden was approximately 20, whereas by 1984 it had increased to some 40. Market forecasts still predict large growth in this area, although CT is expected to face hard competition from magnetic resonance imaging systems (see chapter II.9).

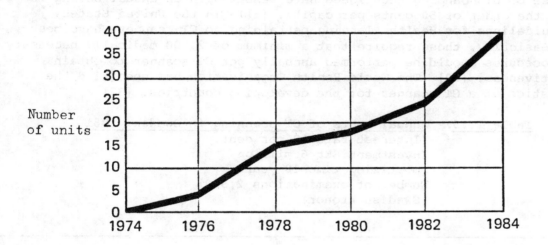

Figure II.12.   Diffusion of CT technology in Sweden

Source: Report on Swedish experiences in DIP.   Prepared
          for the present study by R. Kadefors, 1985.

Available information regarding the efficacy of CT scanning is more conclusive for head than for body scanning. It should be noted also that body scanners are able to perform head scans of equal or superior quality to those produced by head scanners. Several formal policy statements are available on appropriate applications of CT in medical practice. Most of these are from the United States. [28]

Regarding radiation safety, the United States Food and Drug Administration (FDA) has classified CT scanners as class II devices for which technical performance standards are specified. These standards primarily address radiation safety and require information on the imaging performance and radiation dose to be provided to purchasers. Maximum doses received from CT scanners have been found to range from 0.5 rad to 10 rad for a single scan, depending on operating conditions. [29]

Cost-effectiveness

A number of publications are available on the economic evaluation of CT scanning. For Sweden, the costs involved are summarized in table II.5. By adjusting this figure for inflation, it is seen that the cost per examination in Sweden in 1985 was 320 United States dollars. The Swedish study concluded that the use of CT scanning techniques have resulted in an annual saving for society of the order of 50 cents per capita. [31] In the United States, National Guidelines for Health Planning pertaining to CT scanners have been set out. Basically, these require that a minimum of 2,500 medically necessary patient procedures should be performed annually per CT scanner to obtain cost-effectiveness. [30] The World Health Organization has specified the characteristics of a CT scanner for the developing countries. [32]

Table II.5. Annual costs of CT scanning in Sweden, 1981
(Interest rate 12 per cent.
Investment SKr 6 million
Amortizing time 10 years
Number of examinations 2,500)
(Swedish kronor)

Capital	1,062,000	
Remodelling	50,000	
Maintenance	470,000	
Personnel	730,000	
Materials	196,000	
Indirect (administration etc.)	260,000	
Annual total (1981)	2,763,000	(340,000 US dollars)
Average cost per examination (1981)	1,107	(135 US dollars)

Source: Computerized tomography in Sweden. Costs and effects. SPRI, Stockholm, December 1981. In Swedish.

Future of computed tomography

Since the installation of the first CT scanner, the market has undergone great changes both in the number of companies manufacturing CT equipment and in their respective shares of the CT market, resulting in only a few companies on the market.

In the future, CT will compete with the new non-invasive and non-ionizing imaging modalities (ultrasound and MRI). However, its advantages include the fact that it can image bone, which neither MRI nor ultrasound can do.

2.4 Radiotherapy

Operating principle

Surgery, radiotherapy and/or chemotherapy are used for the treatment of cancer. In radiotherapy it is of utmost importance that the radiation dose delivered to the patient should be optimally focused to produce a maximum effect in the volume occupied by the cancerous tissue and a minimal effect in the surrounding healthy tissue. At the same time, certain anatomic areas must be specially protected.

This accuracy requirement has been expressed in performance standards for radiotherapy equipment. [33] Technically, this means that the treatment must be carefully planned, simulated, executed and verified. Treatment planning involves modelling of the absorption characteristics of the radiation (e.g. photons, electrons or protons) within the anatomy of the patient. For modelling, algorithms of varying complexity have been designed. Radiation-beam data is acquired through dosimetry. Patient anatomy is obtained with CT scanners.

To obtain an optimum treatment plan, the cancerous cells are irradiated from several angles and fractioned over a time of approximately two weeks. This sets further requirements for the positioning of the patient for radiotherapy and has led to the present sophisticated simulators and check-and-confirm systems.

Clinical use

It is estimated that the occurrence of cancer will not decrease in the foreseeable future. The available methods to treat the disease are not alternatives but complement each other. The expectations placed on chemotherapy as a general cure for cancer are at present unfounded.

Future of radiotherapy

Radiotherapy utilizes images produced mainly with CT scanners. Planning of therapy needs to be carried out within the true anatomical volume, i.e. in three dimensions (3D). The other trend in radiotherapy deals with the integration of various modules to ensure accurate, reproducible and reliable performance in the radiotherapy clinic.

This concept is being pursued by manufacturers. In the Nordic countries, an R and D programme involving manufacturers, research institutes and users on a precompetition level has been launched to develop next-generation radiotherapy modules and to integrate them via a high-speed network. The programme is called Computer Aided Radiotherapy (CART). The basic concept is illustrated in figure II.13.

3. NUCLEAR MEDICINE

3.1 Gamma camera

Operating principle

Gamma cameras image the photon radiation emitted by radioactive compounds. The technique is based on radioactively-labelled tracers that participate in the metabolism or other body functions and therefore are carried or concentrated in a target organ. Image quality depends on the tracer concentration in the target area and on the emission dynamics of the isotope used.

The imaging detector is made of a NaJ (Tl) crystal, where gamma radiation causes scintillations. These are amplified with photomultipliers and the number of scintillations is counted electronically. Spatial localization of the emitting source is accomplished with a collimator. Image size is 64 x 64 pixels and, with some gamma cameras, even 128 x 128 pixels or 256 x 256 pixels. The dynamic range is 8-10 bits.

The detecting part of the process has changed very little in recent years. Major advances have been made in tracer technology and in image processing. In nuclear medicine the aim is to detect and analyse the physiological or chemical function of target organs. The organs and functions that can be imaged depend on the tracers which are available. The examination is normally done dynamically, resulting in a series of digital images representing the localized time-varying radioactivities. These are then analysed using a mathematical model describing the kinetics, transport mechanisms etc. of the function of the target organ being studied.

The computed tomography principles are also being applied to nuclear medicine, with the single photon emission tomograph (SPET). Single photon emission computed tomography is based on a rotating gamma camera. Whereas in X-ray CT the image is formed using the absorption of X-rays, in SPET the image is reconstructed using the counted number of emitted photons. As with X-ray CT, the first SPET cameras are of the rotating type with rather long scan times. Development efforts are being aimed at reducing this time, e.g. by using a stationary ring.

Major developments in nuclear medicine imaging are shown in figure II.14.

Besides their application in nuclear imaging, isotopes are also used in quantitative analysis in clinical chemistry. Radio-immuno-assay (RIA) was for a long time the only available method of analysing the immune system.

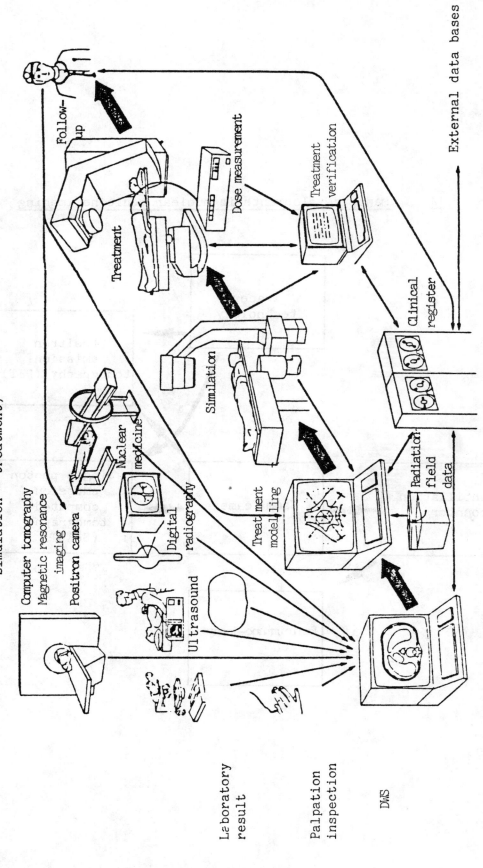

Figure II.13. CART concept of integration of radiotherapy modules (bold arrows indicate principal information flow within the system: image processing – dose planning – simulation – treatment)

Computer tomography
Magnetic resonance imaging
Positron camera
Nuclear medicine
Digital radiography
Ultrasound

Laboratory result

Palpation inspection

DWS

Treatment modelling

Simulation

Treatment

Follow-up

Dose measurement

Treatment verification

Radiation field data

Clinical register

External data bases

Source: CART – Computer aided radiotherapy – Report of the prestudy phase. NORDFORSKs publication series, 1984:1, 73 pages.

Figure II.14.   Major developments in nuclear medicine imaging

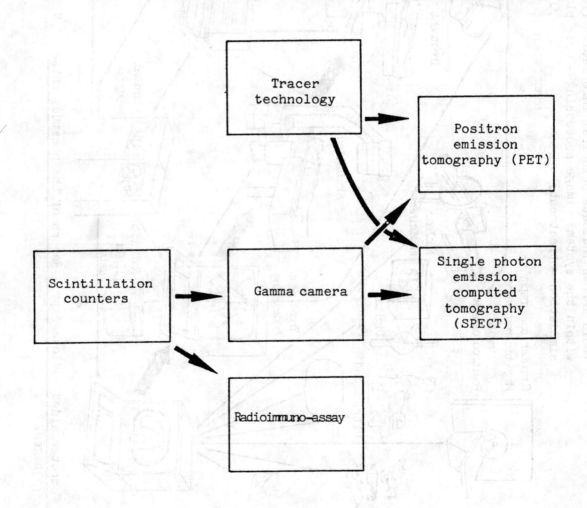

Clinical use

Gamma cameras have been around for nearly 20 years. The largest
application area today is the heart, where thallium-201 and technetium-99
labelled tracers are used to image the cardiac function. Other areas include
the brain, thyroid, kidneys and parathyroid. [34] The clinical applications
are limited by the available tracers. Monoclonal antibodies are expected to
give directions for nuclear medicine in the near future, one of the areas
being the monitoring of chemotherapy in oncology. [35]

Cost-effectiveness

Gamma camera technology is well established and has proved during the
years of its existence to be cost-effective in many applications. It is very
cheap compared with MRI, but uses ionizing radiation for data acquisition.

In the United States, the National Electrical Manufacturers
Association (NEMA) has published a standard that can be used periodically
to control the image quality produced by the gamma camera. [36]

Future of gamma cameras

It can be expected that the gamma-camera technology will be in use for a
long time, since it is extremely useful in imaging the heart function, as well
as other organs. However, the market is not expected to grow.

More and more of the functions of a gamma camera are realized with
software. This creates the need to verify the correct functioning of the
system. A cost project is being started in 1987 in collaboration by
west European countries to develop software phantoms for this purpose.

3.2 Positron-emission tomography

Operating principle

A positron-emission tomography (PET) scanner is a large
computer-controlled tomography unit that maps the distribution of
pharmaceuticals labelled with positron-emitting isotopes in order to construct
detailed images of organ metabolism, physiology and function. Positron
applications are based on the coincidence detection of the two quanta emitted
in opposite directions as a result of the annihilation of the
positron-electron pair (figure II.15). These applications began in the early
1950s. Recent improvements in computer technology have further stimulated
interest in this field, as have developments in the rapid synthesis of a wide
variety of radiopharmaceuticals labelled with short-lived cyclotron-produced
radionuclides. [37] Time-of-flight PET measures the difference in travel
times of the two quanta. This can be used to give the annihilation position.
It requires more efficient detectors and more computing power, however.

Clinical use

Positron-emmission tomography is an analytical imaging technique that
provides a way of making in vivo measurements of the anatomical distribution
and rates of specific biochemical reactions, especially in the brain. [38]

Figure II.15.   Principle of positron-emission tomography
(The quanta are detected with a ring of
detectors feeding data to a computer. The
reconstructed image is displayed on a
screen)

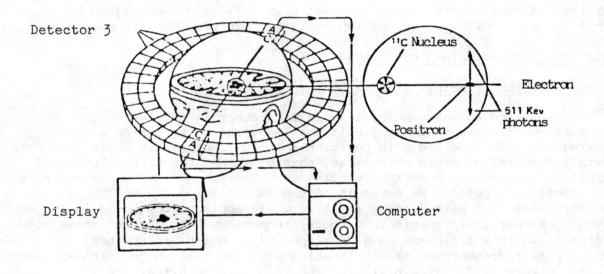

Detector 3

Display

Computer

Source: G. Bergson, et al. Positron emitting organic molecules -
production and use. National Research Council of Sweden,
annual report 1981/82. In Swedish.

The use of PET to obtain these images requires the integration of three components: compounds labelled with radioisotopes, the PET device, and tracer kinetic mathematical models.

The positron emitters mostly used, with their half-lives, are listed in table II.6. They are tagged to various metabolically-active compounds such as glucose, or naturally occurring compounds such as carbon monoxide to image the brain, heart and tumours. The compounds are administered to the patient usually by injection but sometimes also by inhalation. The tracer kinetic models have given rise to much criticism and scepticism, as discussed by Phelps and Mazziotta. [38]

Table II.6. Positron emitters mostly used in positron-emission tomography studies

Isotope	Half-life (minutes)
Carbon-11	20.4
Fluorine-18	110
Oxygen-15	2.05
Nitrogen-13	9.98

Source: R. Dagani, Radiochemicals key to new diagnostic tool. CSEN, 9 November 1981, pp.30-37.

Cost-effectiveness

Positron-emission tomography technology is so new that cost-effectiveness studies have not yet been made.

Future of positron-emission tomography

The central issue in PET today is its cost. It requires a cyclotron facility with the necessary radiopharmaceutical manpower, besides the PET scanner. However, a cyclotron for just the production of positron emitters could be made available at a cost of only $US 250,000. The preparation of the compounds could also be handled by one person. [39] Against this background, the disadvantages of relatively high cost may to a large extent be eliminated.

Positron-emission tomography has potential for imaging the functioning of the brain. However, the technology for making PET images is still developing, its clinical applications have not yet been assessed in full, and there are problems in the kinetic models used. Also, PET will be competing with other imaging modalities.

4.   ULTRASONIC IMAGING

Ultrasonic imaging is not a new technology. It was first used in the clinical practice of obstetrics in 1958 to record foetal heart rate during labour. Its development to the present level of numerous clinical applications and technological capability has been very slow, especially when compared with the immediate success of CT. This is partly due to limitations in available technologies, but a major factor has certainly been that ultrasound has no natural constituency in the medical specialities, and that the images produced by it cannot be readily verified and/or compared with images produced by other modalities.

Operating principle

The application of ultrasound in medicine is based on the sonar principle. Acoustic waves are easily transmitted in water and reflected at interfaces according to the change in the acoustic impedance. Tissue, with the exception of bone and lungs, is mainly composed of water and transmits acoustic waves easily. The key element of the ultrasound imager is the transducer that changes voltage into high-frequency sound by means of a piezo-electric crystal. This crystal is also used to pick up the reflected sound and to convert it into voltage.

Ultrasonic imaging applications have evolved from a simple one-transducer system used to detect, for example, the centreline of the brain (A-mode) to a sophisticated transducer system capable of imaging in real-time in two dimensions and producing cross-sectional images (B-mode) where tissue interfaces (changes in acoustic impedances) are visualized on a grey scale (figure II.16). The principle of a B-mode ultrasound imaging system is illustrated in figure II.17. There are at present several transducer constructions available for B-mode imaging.

The Doppler shift in frequency is widely used to record and monitor blood-flow profiles and velocities. Lately it has been combined with B-mode scanning, making possible the measurement of flow in ultrasound images. This technique can be used, for example, to diagnose coronary stenosis.

Tissue characterization is one of the most interesting future applications of ultrasound. Utilization of the transmitted ultrasound energy to complement the information obtained by reflection may be one way of obtaining this goal.

The contrast and resolution of an ultrasound image are influenced by the ultrasonic frequency. The higher it is, the better the longitudinal resolution, but also the shorter the penetration depth of the pulse. This means that, to achieve the required penetration, a lower frequency must be used than would be desirable from the point of view of good resolution. The frequencies used range from 1 to 15 MHz. The volume that the transducer sees in focus depends on the transducer construction.

The ultrasound image can easily be converted into a digital form. Image-processing algorithms are used for averaging images before display or for deconvolution to enhance edges. The image at present consists of a maximum of 512 x 512 pixels or in polar co-ordinates of 256 lines x 512 pixels. The dynamic range is 4-8 bits.

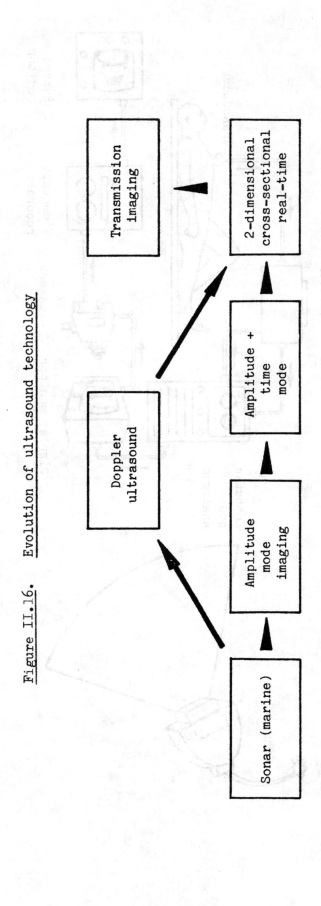

Figure II.16. Evolution of ultrasound technology

Source: Office of Technology Assessment, US Congress, Policy Implications of the Computed Tomography (CT) Scanner, GPO Stock No.052-003-00565-4, Washington D.C. US Governmental Printing Office, August 1978, p.68.

- 47 -

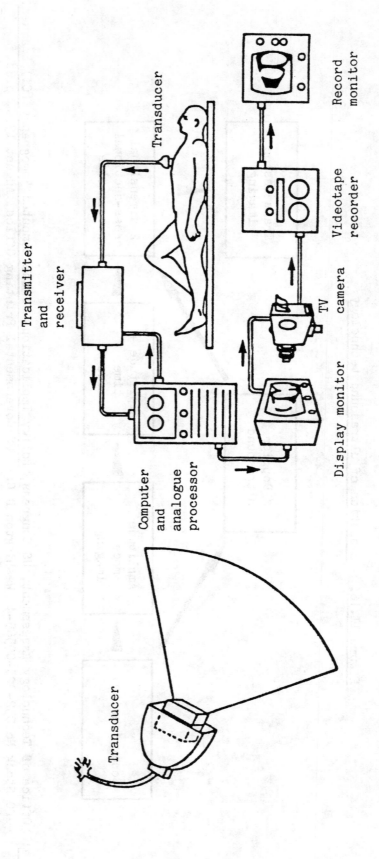

Figure II.17. Schematic block diagram of a B-mode ultrasound imaging system

Source: Office of Technology Assessment, US Congress, Policy Implications of the Computed Tomography (CT) Scanner, GPO Stock No.052-003-00565-4, Washington D.C. US Governmental Printing Office, August 1978, p.68.

- 48 -

Clinical use

In addition to its use in obstetrics, applications have expanded to include studies of the heart, brain, eyes and various organs and structures of the abdomen (including the liver, gall bladder, spleen, pancreas, kidneys and adrenal glands). The medical specialities using ultrasound technology are shown in table II.7.

Table II.7. Distribution of ultrasound systems between medical specialities (based on the sales of systems to some European countries in 1984)

Segment	Revenue		Sales	
	Million US dollars	Percentage	Units	Percentage
Cardiology	47.7	26.6	746	13.0
Radiology	58.0	32.3	1 585	27.6
Obstetrics	48.2	26.9	1 610	28.0
Misc. hospital	5.8	3.2	230	4.0
All private	19.8	11.0	1 575	27.4
Total	179.5	100	5 746	100

Source: Biomedical Business International, vol.VIII, 1985, p.158.

Unlike the other imaging modalities, ultrasound is utilized in several medical specialities, as shown in table II.7. This is due to the way this technology has diffused into medicine. Its main advocates have been physicians rather than radiologists.

The other reason for this pattern is that the energies involved in diagnostic ultrasound are generally believed to be safe. However, it has not been conclusively shown that no risks are involved. Therefore it is more realistic to say that the risk associated with ultrasonic energy is unknown rather than non-existent. An indication of that concern is the consensus statement issued by the seminar recently organized by the National Institute of Health (NIH) in the United States on the use of diagnostic ultrasound in pregnancy, which recommended that the use of ultrasound should be restricted to those cases where its use could be justified by clinical indications. This would mean that the technology should not be used as a routine screening method in pregnancy. [40]

At present there are almost 100 different models of B-mode ultrasound scanners on the market. Comparison of their technical performance is not readily possible owing to lack of international performance standards. This was also the reason for the publication, in 1986, by the IEC Sub-Committee 29D "Ultrasonics" of its standard on methods of measuring the performance of

ultrasonic pulse-echo diagnostic equipment. [41] Several working groups of
the IEC/SC 29D are currently engaged in work on other related subjects. [42]
As an example of a national approach in this field, the recently issued USSR
(GOST) standard on ultrasound diagnostic equipment can be mentioned. [43]

Image quality can be measured by the users using image phantoms. More
complete measurements of the imaging qualities require special instrumentation.

Cost-effectiveness

In addition to the safety aspect, ultrasound equipment is much less
expensive than CT or MRI scanners. The prices range from $US 10,000 to
$US 150,000. A real-time B-mode scanner costs approximately $50,000. They
are small, have no special installation requirements and are portable.

The cost per examination depends on the use of the equipment. Assuming
an amortization period of five years for a $50,000 scanner and
1,500 examinations annually, the break-even cost is approximately $30. [44]

Future of ultrasound

Because ultrasound is non-invasive, considered to be safe, easy to use
and relatively cheap, its utilization is at present already very wide. It
will continue to grow within the next few years (see also table II.8). The
World Health Organization has produced guidelines for ultrasonic equipment
intended for use in the developing countries, pointing to a wider diffusion of
this technology. [45]

Table II.8. Selected producers and suppliers of medical
ultrasound equipment, 1985-1987

Company	Unit sales by year		
	1985	1986	1987
Diasonics	325	375	425
ATL	250	300	330
GE	300	325	355
Philips	240	240	245
Acuson	210	240	270
Toshiba	70	80	90
Siemens	50	60	70

Source: Diagnostic Imaging, 1986 (Original source:
Hambrecht and Quist, San Francisco).

5. MAGNETIC RESONANCE IMAGING

Introduction

Magnetic resonance imaging (MRI, also called nuclear magnetic resonance, NMR) is a new diagnostic imaging modality that has aroused a wide interest for a number of reasons. First, it employs radio waves and magnetic fields, eliminating the risk of ionizing irradiation. Secondly, in addition to providing very good distinction between adjacent structures, it affords excellent tissue contrast without the need for injection of potentially toxic contrast agents. Thirdly, with MRI, bone does not interfere with the signal providing visualization of areas, such as the posterior fossa, brain stem and spinal cord, that previously could not be imaged non-invasively. Fourthly, and potentially of greatest importance, it offers the possibility of detecting diseases at earlier stages than previously because MRI is sensitive to the physical and chemical characteristics of cells. [46]

However, the MRI imagers are at present expensive and their installation is costly. MRI requires more physician time in patient examinations than other already-established techniques. Moreover, the exact role of MRI in clinical medicine, particularly its efficacy compared with other imaging modalities, has not yet been determined.

The technology is diffusing very rapidly despite these concerns. In January 1983, 14 MRI units were installed in the United States. By October 1983, the number had increased to 34 and by August 1984 there were 93 units in the United States, and at least 145 in the world. [46] More recent data on MRI installations in the United States may be found in chapter V.

Operating principle

The existence of the nuclear magnetic resonance phenomenon was first demonstrated in 1946 by Block and Purcell, who in 1952 received the Nobel Prize for Physics for their discovery. The first magnetic resonance image (of two tubes of water) was published by Lauterbur in 1973. The nuclear magnetic resonance phenomenon relates to the nuclei (protons and neutrons) of atoms. Those nuclei that contain an odd number of protons or neutrons have an intrinsic angular momentum, called "spin". Since nuclei are electrically charged, the nuclei that spin produce a magnetic field. Only those nuclei that are magnetic can be used in MRI.

Supplying electromagnetic energy at the appropriate rotational frequency will excite the nuclei from a lower energy level, E_1, to a higher level, E_2. If the energy is turned off, the excited nuclei drop back to level E_1 (relax) and in so doing emit the energy they absorbed in moving from E_1 to E_2. If the energy is repeatedly applied the nuclei will resonate between E_1 and E_2.

Since the emitted signals are extremely weak, atoms must be present in sufficient concentration in order to produce a strong enough signal for MRI purposes. To date, the atom most commonly used has been hydrogen. The imaging of sodium and phosphorus would also be of great interest but requires more sophistication of the technologies involved.

The signal produced is not only proportional to hydrogen density, but depends on the velocity with which fluid is flowing through the structure being imaged. It is also affected by the rate at which the excited nuclei relax. These relaxation parameters are marked T_1 and T_2. The extent to which a magnetic resonance image reflects each of these four parameters (nuclei density, flow, T_1 and T_2) depends on the electromagnetic pulse sequence employed to excite the nuclei in the region being imaged. Therefore there is no such thing as a "unique" magnetic resonance image. Rather, the images vary according to the pulse sequence used. [46]

Spatial encoding of the MRI signals is accomplished by applying a magnetic field gradient across the region of interest. An external magnetic field will change the rotational frequency of nuclei. Therefore when the energy pulse is applied, only those nuclei resonate that have the same rotational frequency. By sequentially varying the frequency of the energy being supplied, nuclei can be selectively excited. Several techniques have been developed whereby MRI information can be spatially encoded, acquired and transformed into an image. One of these is electronically to rotate the magnetic field gradients to obtain multiple projections that a computer can piece together to construct a magnetic resonance image. Newer techniques are more efficient with regard to the scan-time required, approaching scan-times of the order of milliseconds.

The components necessary for producing a magnetic resonance image (figure II.18) include: (i) a magnet with a large enough aperture to enclose the structure being imaged. The magnet is used to produce a highly uniform magnetic field within the structure being imaged; (ii) gradient coils to create the magnetic field gradient required for spatial encoding of the MRI signals; (iii) a transmitter operating at radio-frequencies to produce the pulse sequence to resonate the nuclei; (iv) a receiver to detect the MRI signals emitted during relaxation; (v) a computer and display to control system operation and to reconstruct, store and display the image; and (vi) the homogeneity of the field can be corrected with shim coils that are suitably placed (figure II.18).

Magnets

Although nuclear magnetic resonance spectroscopy had existed for many years, magnets with large enough apertures for human imaging became available only after interest in MRI emerged. It must be noted that the price of the magnet is the main cause of the high purchasing and installation costs of MRI scanners. Technically, MRI magnets are characterized by magnet type, field strength, aperture size and field homogeneity.

The static magnetic field can be produced with electromagnets (resistive or superconductive) or permanent magnets. Resistive magnets require energy and cooling and have a limited field strength (approx. 0.2 Tesla). Superconductive magnets provide large field strengths that are highly stable and uniform. They require a cooling system of liquid helium and liquid nitrogen. Both types suffer from sensitivity to external magnetic objects and produce large fringe fields. For these reasons, preventive installation-site preparation is necessary. Permanent magnets do not have these problems. They are, however, extremely heavy (as much as 100 tonnes) and have a limited field strength (approx. 0.3 Tesla). [47]

Field strength is a topic of much controversy. Theoretically, a higher field strength results in a better signal-to-noise ratio. However, it is unclear above which level image quality ceases to improve. At the moment, the marketed MRI scanners have field strengths of from 0.15 to 2 Tesla (table II.9).

Clinical use

To date, since adequate precautions have been taken, no significant biological risks associated with the use of MRI have been identified. The clinical imaging applications in which most experience has been gained are imaging of the brain and of the central nervous system. Results with the heart and pelvis are also promising. The scope of the role of MRI in medicine is yet to be determined, however.

Markets

In 1985 there were 26 companies that marketed or intended to market MRI scanners (table II.9). Comparing this with the development of CT scanner markets (18 originally, 10 remaining), it is improbable that all will survive.

Projections for the growth of this market are very favourable (table II.10). Despite its potential, it is expected that the proliferation of MRI technology will be slower than that of the CT scanners, because:

(i)   Considerable research is still necessary to prove its clinical efficacy in applications;

(ii) Unit system costs are high;

(iii) Life-cycles for the first generation of MRI scanners are short, owing to new technological developments making them obsolete; and

(iv) Those responsible for providing health care will be cautious in investing in this technology.

Figure II.18.

The components of a magnetic resonance imaging system

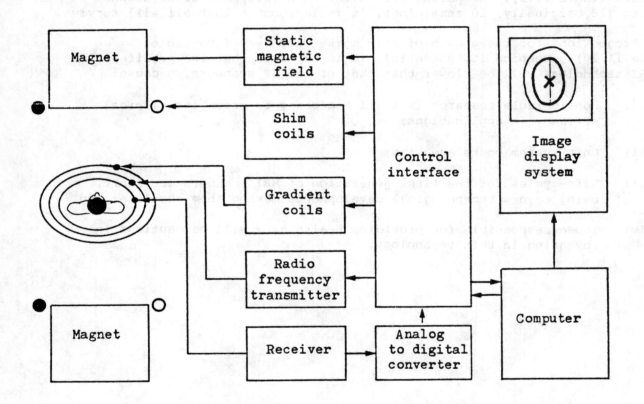

Source: Health Technology Case Study 27. Nuclear Magnetic Resonance Imaging Technology: A clinical, Industrial and Policy Analysis. Washington, DC. US Congress Office of Technology Assessment, OTA-HCS-27, September 1984, p.20.

Table II.9. Companies producing magnetic resonance imaging systems

Company	Product
DVANCED NMR SYSTEMS	High-field (4T) small-bore magnet for scientific applications under development
NSALDO BIOMEDICAL LECTRONICS	System under development
SAHI CHEMICAL	0.1T resistive system and superconducting system under development
RUKER INSTRUMENTS	0.15T and 0.3T resistive systems with integral iron magnetic shielding
GR	0.5T superconducting system available
IASONICS	0.35T superconducting system available
LSCINT	0.35T and 0.5T superconducting systems available, low-cost 2.0T system in development
IELD EFFECTS	Permanent magnet system in development
ONAR	0.3T permanent magnet system available 0.3T resistive mobile system available
.E. MEDICAL SYSTEMS DIV.	1.5T superconducting system available
OLD STAR INDUSTRIES	Low-cost ($500,000) resistive system available, not marketed in the United States
ITACHI	0.15T resistive system and superconducting in development
BM INSTRUMENTS	System under development
NSTRUMENTARIUM	Low-field (0.02T), low-cost resistive system
ITSUBISHI ELECTRIC	0.6T superconductive system using a 1.5T magnet
& D TECHNOLOGY	0.15T resistive system with transverse field available
ALORAC CRYOGENICS	Small-bore, high-field paediatric unit under development
MR IMAGING	Low-cost head system using permanent magnet
HILIPS	0.5T and 1.5T systems available on limited basis
ICKER INTL	0.15T resistive system available 0.5T, 1.0T, 1.5T, 2.0T superconducting systems available
ESONEX	Resistive and permanent magnet systems for cardiac studies
AWYO ELECTRIC	System under development
HIMADZU	0.15T resistive system in evaluation
IEMENS	0.5T, 1.0T, 1.5T, 2.0T superconducting systems available
ECHNICARE	0.15T resistive system available 0.6T, 1.5T superconducting system available
OSHIBA	0.15T resistive system available Superconducting system under development

Source: Biomedical Business International, vol. VIII, 1985, p. 139.

Table II.10. Projected world-wide market for
magnetic resonance imaging systems

Year	Annual unit deliveries	Cumulative unit deliveries	Average sales price per system (US dollars)	Total annual sales (million US dollars)
1982	15	15	1 300 000	20
1983*	75	90	1 300 000	100
1984*	200	290	1 500 000	300
1985*	400	690	1 600 000	650
1986*	650	1 340	1 700 000	1 100
1987*	950	2 290	1 850 000	1 750
1988*	1 250	3 540	2 000 000	2 500

Source: Health Technology Case Study 27. Nuclear Magnetic Resonance
Imaging Technology: A Clinical, Industrial and Policy Analysis.
Washington, DC. United States Congress Office of Technology Assessment,
OTA-HCS-27, September 1984, p.58.

Cost-effectiveness

At this moment, no complete cost studies for MRI are available.
Furthermore, the technology and the protocols according to which it is applied
in medicine are developing rapidly, making such studies obsolete in a short
time. However, the OTA Study on MRI has estimated the costs per examination
to be between $US 121 and $US 382. [48] These figures are based on the
various MRI systems available and costs related to their installation.
Operating costs include energy, personnel, supplies and maintenance.
Overheads that include administration, building, etc. are estimated at
25 per cent of operating costs. The purchasing cost is amortized over five
years with a 10 per cent interest rate. The facility modification costs are
amortized over 10 years at a 10 per cent interest rate. A later study by
Evens [49] arrived at a much higher break-even cost of $1,100 in comparable
circumstances. The annual costs were estimated at approximately $900,000.

In figure II.19, a possible approach to a break-even analysis is
presented. It is estimated that one MRI examination takes 1 to 1.5 hours. In
single shifts, only five patients per day can be examined. A better solution
is achieved if work is done in two shifts. This of course increases the
personnel costs. However, given the high proportion of fixed costs, it is of
great economic importance to increase the utilization of this system.

Figure II.19. Break-even analysis for various
MRI systems

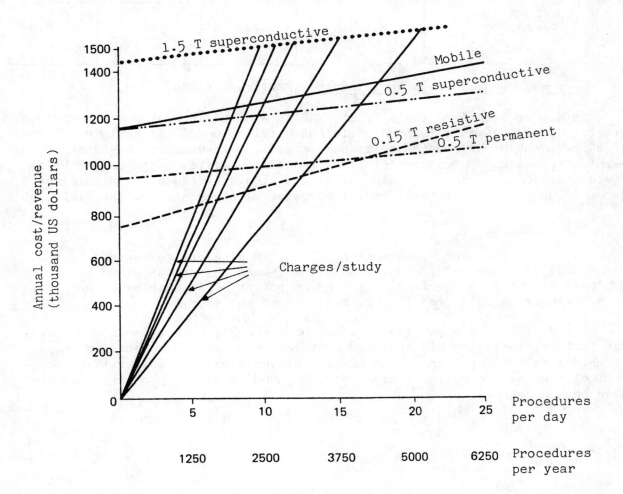

Source: Medical Engineering Laboratory,
Technical Research Centre of Finland (based on United States'
sources).

Table II.11. Approximate annual costs of various
types of MRI equipment
(Millions of Swedish kronor)

Equipment and size of investment	Semi-permanent magnet	Resistive low-field magnet	Resistive magnet	Supercon-ductive magnet
Purchase cost	10.0	3.5	9.0	12.0
Annual capital cost	2.5	0.9	2.4	3.1
Annual operational cost	1.9	1.3	2.0	2.3
Total Annual Cost	4.4	2.2	4.4	5.4

Source: Magnetic Resonance Imaging, SPRI report 206.

As may be seen from table II.11, MRI is a costly process. This obviously creates special demands for the efficient utilization of the equipment. Some 70-80 per cent of MRI costs are fixed costs, i.e. they are independent of examination volume. Examples of fixed costs are capital costs and certain operational costs such as liquid helium and liquid nitrogen. Variable costs (some 20-30 per cent of total costs) comprise mainly staff and material. [50]

Future of MRI

The advantages and disadvantages of MRI imaging are summarized in the OTA Study. [51] However, considerably more research, as described in table II.12, will be required before MRI's potential is determined and its most appropriate roles in clinical medicine established.

The decision of a manufacturer to enter the MRI market depends on several key factors, including his ability to attract capital and scientific or technical talent for R and D, to develop strong ties with universities and medical centres for collaborative research, and to market products once they have been developed.

Table II.12. Likely areas for future research
in magnetic resonance imaging

---

1. Determination of clinical utility of MRI compared with other imaging modalities

2. Improvements in magnet design (e.g. increased field uniformity, increased field strength, techniques for conserving liquid helium and nitrogen)

3. Determination of magnetic field strength that yields optimum image quality for hydrogen and other nuclei

4. Identification of pulse sequence optimum for demonstrating various types of pathologies

5. Improvements in imaging software and techniques affecting image quality, resolution, and scan time

6. Optimization of radio-frequency coils

7. Development of new and improved surface coils

8. Improvements in siting and shielding techniques

9. Development of paramagnetic agents for assessing tissue pathophysiology

10. Further development of whole-body spectroscopic techniques and applications

11. Imaging of nuclei other than hydrogen (e.g. sodium or phosphorus)

Source: Health Technology Case Study 27. Nuclear Magnetic Resonance
Imaging Technology: A Clinical, Industrial and Policy Analysis.
Washington, D.C. United States Congress Office of Technology Assessment,
OTA-HCS-27, September 1984, p.32.

6.   DIGITAL X-RAY FILMS

X-ray films can be digitized with many techniques of varying degrees of accuracy and speed. High resolution CCD line arrays (CCD = charge-coupled-device) are one promising solution with enough spatial resolution and speed (e.g. 2048 elements).

7.   OTHER MEDICAL APPLICATIONS

At the moment, the emphasis in imaging in clinical medicine is on the modalities discussed in the previous sections of this chapter. However, microscopy and especially cell analysis has also been a topic of active DI R and D efforts for several years.

Cardiac imaging

In some areas of diagnostic imaging, image processing has played a very important role. These applications have dealt mainly with the imaging of the heart function and anatomy. Fluoroscopic techniques with video recording and cine cameras and B-mode ultrasound have been used to acquire functional images of the heart. These images, having been digitized, are processed by algorithms, to produce 3D representations of the functioning of the left ventricle of the heart and of wall motion. Coronary arteries can also be visualized in 3D with these techniques. An excellent overview of the present situation making possible the localization and assessment of stenosis has been written by M. Kuwahara. [52]

Images produced with gamma cameras using thallium and technetium labelled agents are also used to image the heart function.

All the above-mentioned methods are able to image the heart function dynamically. Quantitative indices of the heart function can also be computed from these image sequences.

Chromosome analysis [53]

In chromosome analysis, DI may be used both to automate the time-consuming and boring work of locating cells in metaphase that can be analysed and to help in the interactive karyotyping of the cells. There are at least two products on the market claiming to solve these problems: Magiscan from Joyce-Loebl and IBAS 2 from Kontron, both equipped with suitable software. As in the case of the haematology systems, these first-generation products have questionable price/performance. But new products are forthcoming. The Swedish company IMTEC - Image Technology AB is involved in the final testing stages of an automated metaphase finder and interactive karyotyping system that it hopes to put on the market very soon. The system should have a performance that makes it quite useful. There is reason to believe that other companies have new models under preparation.

Cytology [53]

Research in DI as applied to cytology has been going on since the early 1960s. The main application has been aimed at automating the screening for cervical cancer by looking at smears from the uterine cervix. Since these screening programmes involve many millions of samples every year and occupy several thousand laboratory technicians with simple routine work, the motives for automation are strong. But the difficulties in this field are great and several early systems have failed to meet expectations. In this field also, the development in technology makes it likely that useful solutions will appear soon. IMTEC has been working in this field since 1973 and has finally developed a system which could work. The methods have been tested on several hundred patient samples and found to work as well as visual screening. A clinical prototype developed by IMTEC was tested in 1986. Other companies, such as Shandon, Leitz and Kontron, are also reporting progress in this area. In Japan, a national cancer programme has just started and will spend several million dollars per year in an attempt to develop a good solution to this problem. It is to be hoped that these systems will mean the first massive, successful use of fully automated image analysis in medicine.

In cytology, the interest in interactive systems is increasing, i.e. systems similar to the work-stations in radiology. These systems are used for the study of the manner in which cell populations are affected by malignant processes. There are strong indications that such studies can provide information of prognostic value that may influence the treatment of a cancer patient.

Haematology

For the diagnosis and treatment of certain diseases, the types and numbers of white blood cells (leukocytes) present in the circulation are important. With a healthy individual, the types and numbers of leukocytes are within certain limits. When disease is present, the numbers can change dramatically and new types can enter the circulation. In clinical routine, these are measured manually with a microscope. In a manual technique the number of cells that can be counted is limited to 100-200, resulting in a large statistical error probability. Although attempts have been made since the beginning of the 1970s to automate this procedure, there has as yet been no real breakthrough. Some products have reached the market, but so far they have not been generally accepted by the users. The potential need for an automated white-blood-cell analyser is large, providing it is reliable, fast and inexpensive.

Owing to limitations in available computer technology (computing power/price) these requirements cannot be met at present. The algorithms necessary for cell identification require colour images and are very complex, necessitating a large computer. However, the advances in VLSI and array processors with the resulting improved performance/cost ratio should make these products more competitive in the near future.

Clinical chemistry

Many procedures in clinical chemistry are based on the detection of changes in the optical properties of the samples when a specific reaction is taking place (kinetic measurement) or when the reaction is completed (end-point measurement). Fibre optics and high resolution CCD-cameras are at present being used to develop new applications.

Thermography

Thermography is based on the imaging of the infrared radiation (heat) emitted by the body. The imagers have been on the market for many years, but the technology has not been widely accepted, despite its relatively low cost. Its clinical uses are restricted to cases where there is a locally hot/cold spot on the skin or very close to the skin. Detection of breast cancer has been one advocated application, but thermography has not succeeded in replacing conventional X-ray mammography.

8.   PICTURE ARCHIVING AND COMMUNICATION SYSTEMS

8.1   Introduction

Integration of medical imaging devices and image processing facilities will result in a picture archiving and communication system (PACS) as presented in figure II.1. Owing to the gradual transfer from non-digital imaging devices to digital ones and the continuous refinement of technologies behind PACS, PACS will not be adopted as a total system, but rather grow piece by piece.

The main components of PACS are illustrated in figure II.20. The imaging devices communicate the acquired images through the network using a standardized transmission protocol. The images may be compressed to decrease the transmission time. Digital images are stored on a medium capable of storing a large number of images in a read-only fashion (the information cannot be electrically erased) using a data-base system to retrieve the images. Images are viewed on the medical work-stations. When necessary, algorithms can be applied to them to enhance certain features and/or to interpret their clinical information content. Reports and comments can be attached to the images. The station is able to display several images simultaneously. The images and reports are communicated to the referring physicians at the image display stations (see figure II.1). Image hard copies and paper print-outs are available, for example through laser printers.

8.2   Archiving

Storage requirements

Most of the imaging devices sold today produce digital images. However, since the old systems will continue to be used for a long time, some of the images will be available on film only. An example of the situation in 1982 is given in table II.13, showing how the number of examinations and images was divided at the Mallincrodt Institute of Radiology. Table II.13 illustrates clearly how the digital technique will influence the functioning of the imaging department. Although only 10 per cent of the examinations are digital, over 50 per cent of the images are digital, indicating that more images per examination will be taken with the new techniques. A newer study by SPRI indicates that the percentages for digital and film-based examinations are 15/85 per cent. [23]

Figure II.20.   **Main components of a picture archiving
and communication system**

```
┌─────────────────┐   ┌─────────────────┐   ┌─────────────────┐
│  Communication  │   │   Archiving     │   │ Image processing│
│ - Network       │   │ - Data base     │   │ - Display       │
│ - Transmission  │   │ - Storage media │   │ - User interface│
│   protocol      │   │                 │   │ - IP algorithms │
│ - Image format  │   │                 │   │                 │
└────────┬────────┘   └────────┬────────┘   └────────┬────────┘
         │                     │                     │
         └─────────────────────┼─────────────────────┘
                               │
┌──────────────────────────────────────────────────────────────┐
│        Picture Archiving and Communication Systems            │
└──────────────────────────────────────────────────────────────┘
```

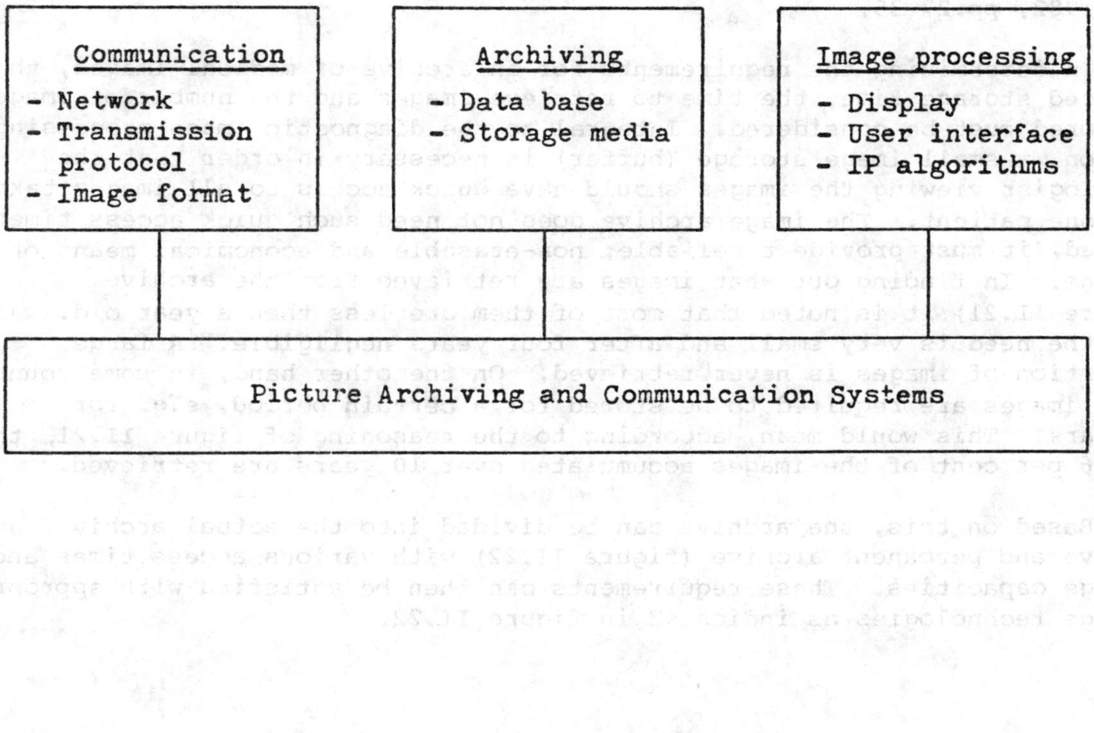

An example (case) illustrating the structure of DI examinations at one advanced hospital is presented in chapter V (Federal Republic of Germany).

Table II.13. Number of examinations and images, digital or film-based at Mallincrodt Institute of Radiology in 1982
(Percentage)

	Examinations	Images
Digital	10.6	53.4
Film	89.4	46.6
Total	100.0	100.0

Source: W. Pratt, "Digital Image Processing". Diagnostic Imaging, July 1982, pp.27-35.

In determining the requirements for an archive of medical images, the required storage time, the time to retrieve images and the number of images to be stored must be considered. Integral to the diagnostic image processing station, a small image storage (buffer) is necessary in order that the radiologist viewing the images should have quick access to all images taken from one patient. The image archive does not need such quick access times. Instead, it must provide a reliable, non-erasable and economical means of storage. In finding out what images are retrieved from the archive (figure II.21) it is noted that most of them are less than a year old. After this the need is very small and after four years negligible. A large proportion of images is never retrieved. On the other hand, in some countries X-ray images are required to be stored for a certain period, e.g. for 10 years. This would mean, according to the reasoning of figure II.21, that only 6 per cent of the images accumulated over 10 years are retrieved.

Based on this, the archive can be divided into the actual archive, active archive and permanent archive (figure II.22) with various access times and storage capacities. These requirements can then be satisfied with appropriate storage technologies as indicated in figure II.22.

Percentage of
X-ray pictures
requested

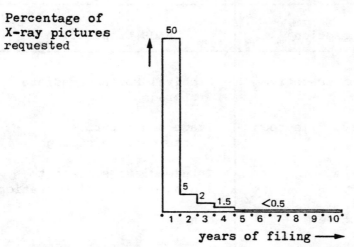

years of filing ⟶

Source: D. Meyer-Ebrecht and T. Wendler, "An architectural route through
PACS." Computer, vol. 16, No.8, pp.19-28.

Figure II.22. A hierarchical archiving system

Storage function

I. Local processor
II. Local operational
storage
III. Picture base buffer
IV. Actual archive
V. Active archive
VI. Permanent archive

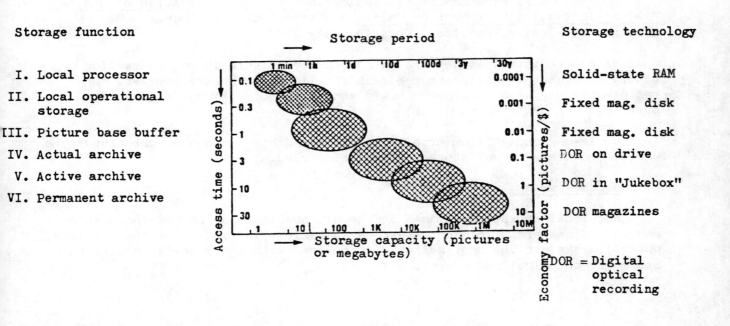

Storage technology

Solid-state RAM
Fixed mag. disk
Fixed mag. disk
DOR on drive
DOR in "Jukebox"
DOR magazines

DOR = Digital
optical
recording

Source: As for figure II.21.

In order to estimate the image transactions in PACS, transactions in the film library system were studied. Some film library transactions will have corresponding image transactions in PACS, others will not. A list of these library transactions and their corresponding PACS transactions is presented in table II.14.

Table II.14. Comparison of film library and picture archiving
and communication systems transactions

Film library transaction	PACS transaction
Inactive file-room to active file-room	Archival to intermediate storage
New films to active file-room	Image generators to intermediate storage
Active file-room to viewstation	Intermediate storage to diagnostic review station
Viewstation to active file-room	None a/
Active file-room to inactive file-room	Movement of new images from intermediate to archival storage b/
Active file-room to borrowers	Intermediate storage to remote display
Borrowers to active file-room	None

Source: M.F. Drummond et al. Guidelines for the Evaluation of Digital Diagnostic Imaging Equipment or Units, Department of Radiology, McMaster University, Hamilton, Ontario, July 1983.

a/ Since digital images are not "returned", there is no transaction similar to returning films to the film room. Occasionally, however, the radiologist may wish to store a newly made transformed image or annotated overlay.

b/ Images copied from archival to intermediate storage do not have to be copied back to archival storage after being used.

Storage media

For local storage of images at the diagnostic image processing station, magnetic disks are at present the most suitable solution. For the archives, optical disks are the most suitable. Compared with the magnetic media, they are more economical and non-erasable [54].

Data-base management

At present, film archives are centralized. With the PACS concept a central question will concern the degree to which the archives should be decentralized. The basic alternatives are either to archive them locally at the imaging device or to have a central archive. In both cases, all images need to be accessible from all diagnostic work-stations.

A centralized data-base management system and the related hardware must be extremely reliable, since all PACS functions require access to the image archive. In addition, because of the large amount of data (of the order 10^{14} bit) that is stored and because of the large number of users that want to retrieve images, the system will be quite complex, as illustrated by figure II.23.

8.3 Communication

Image transfers

At present, diagnostic imaging takes place upon the request of the referring physician. This request contains information about the earlier illnesses and therapies of the patient, the reasons for making the imaging request and the suspected diagnosis. When the images are available, they are transferred to the referring physician in at least three possible ways:

- In emergencies the images are sent immediately and the report will follow later;

- Usually the images and the report are received the following day; or

- In certain cases, consultations are held with the referring physicians to discuss diagnosis and therapy.

A PACS must accommodate these routines to be acceptable.

Transmission

A large number of methods are available for transferring images electrically. Inside the hospital, local area networks (LAN) would be a good solution. However, even the fastest commercially available LANs today are able to transfer data from disk to disk at an effective speed of only 1 Mbps. The transmission of a single CT image (512 x 512 pixel x 12 bit = 3 Mbit) would require 3 s, which is an unacceptably long time. One way to alleviate this problem is to code the image with a compression algorithm so that the amount of bits to be transmitted is smaller. Compressed images must then be reconstructed at the receiving end. This requires additional sophistication from the system. To compensate for errors introduced during transmission, the compression and decompression algorithms incorporate error detection and correction.

The throughput rates of a radiology department LAN have been estimated by the Kansas City PACS group. It is estimated that at that department 13.9 GBytes must be retrieved daily. Assuming a 12-hour working day (overhead time, protocol and a realistic view of LAN software, etc.), the throughput

Figure II.23. Schematic diagram for a large image data-base system

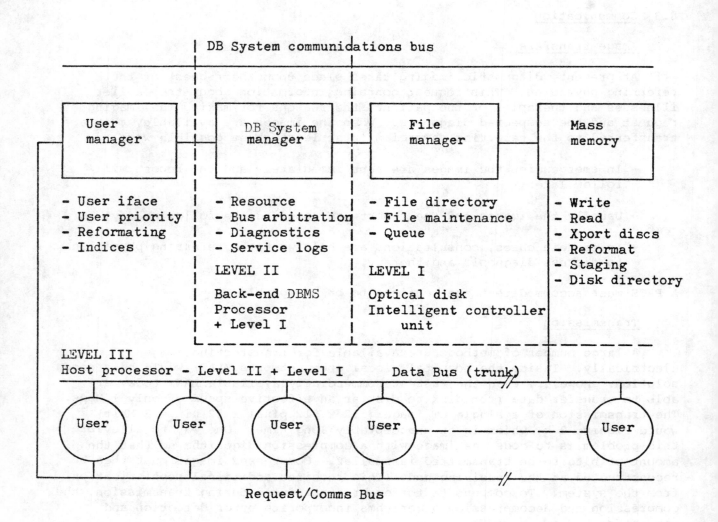

Source: R. Colby, et al., "Promising rapid access high-capacity mass-storage
        technique for diagnostic information utilizing optical disk".
        A. Duerinckx (Ed), PACS I, Proceedings of SPIE, vol. 318, 1982, pp.36-42.

rate requirement is 25.7 Mb/s. This is the upper limit. With a more efficient network protocol, this can be reduced to 11.9 Mb/s. This is still well above the capabilities of current commercial LANs. [55]

Local area networks based on optical fibres will have sufficient band widths to meet the requirements of PACS in a large or medium-scale hospital. This technology is just becoming commercially available.

Image format and communication protocols

Major problems in PACS are the lack of an internationally-accepted standard to code the images for transmission and the lack of a communication protocol for such coded images. The lack of communication protocols is not specific to medical applications only. In fact, it is a major problem in information technology, only recently acknowledged. Consequently, those companies that produce the complete spectrum (or almost) of medical imaging devices are in a better position to offer PACS than companies with only one imaging modality, since they know how to interconnect their products. However, since most of the companies use computer hardware that is not produced by them, all would in the end benefit from a common communication protocol.

Probably the most appropriate communication protocol would be OSI (open systems interconnection), which is being developed by ISO (International Organization for Standardization) and is receiving support from the major computer manufacturers and national standardization organizations. The American College of Radiology (ACR) together with the National Electrical Manufacturers Association (NEMA) has prepared a standard for image format and for a communication protocol for medical images. The communication protocol is based on the OSI layers and utilizes the four lowest of the seven OSI layers. A technical description of the communication is shown schematically in figure II.24. A further discussion of this and the image format standard may be found in chapter VI.1.

8.4 Image work-station

Role of image work-stations

In a film-based X-ray department, the radiologist dictates his report by viewing the X-ray films presented to him with a lightbox. The referring physician in turn views the images with a lightbox. In the digital system, image work-stations form the interface between the PACS and the users. They are used to display the images the user recalls to the screen by means of the commands available. The complexity of the work-station can range from a simple display station to a diagnostic work-station able to manipulate and visualize 3D images.

Performance requirements

Some of the principal requirements for the performance of a diagnostic work-station (DWS) are as follows: the stations must be easily accessible, placed at convenient locations, either centralized at an "image bar" or distributed to the physicians' rooms; all images must be accessible equally easily (retrieval of sequential images and images related to the same patient

Figure II.24.   Summary of protocol layers for ACR-NEMA standard
and for OSI

Location of
ACR-NEMA
interface plane

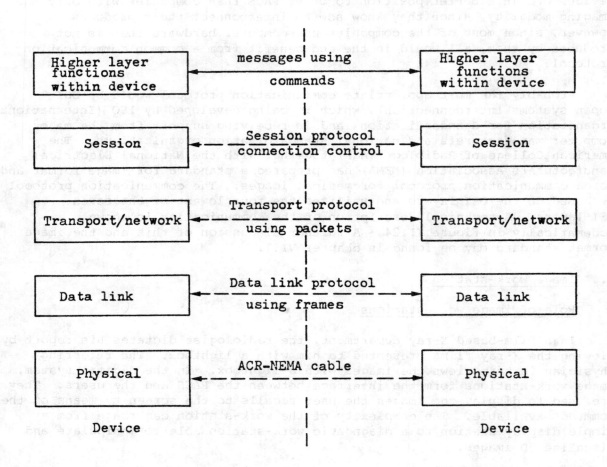

Source: ACR-NEMA Digital Imaging and Communications Standard,
1 July 1985.

must be especially easy and quick); retrieval times in general should be short, in order that the PACS should not be less efficient than the conventional method; DWS should be able to display several images simultaneously, either on one large screen or on several separate screens; the size of the display should be suitable for viewing also in physician consultation sessions.

The information content of images varies depending on the image source. The highest requirement is set by thorax X-ray images for which a resolution of 4,000 x 4,000 pixel with 12 bit dynamic range may even be necessary. With windowing and zooming, the screen resolution of DWS can be decreased to 1,000 x 1,000 pixel, which is a manageable figure with present techniques.

A broad variety of image-processing algorithms are necessary. These include selection of the dynamic range for display (windowing), filtering to remove distortion caused by the imaging device and image enhancement to emphasize image detail. Additional operations include subtraction and reconstruction of images from selected projection and calculation of quantitative data from the images (e.g. volumes and flows). The possibility of manipulating and processing images is one of the most important advantages offered by digital technology. A suggestion for the sequencing of these operations is given in figure II.25.

It is essential for DWS to be able also to handle and display data other than images, such as strings and one-dimensional signals. These must be flexibly integrated into the image data base.

Structure of DWS

The resolution and dynamic range requirements for a DWS originate from the performance capabilities of medical imaging devices (table II.15).

Table II.15. Spatial resolution and dynamic range of
medical imagining devices
(potential values in parentheses)

	Resolution /pixel	Dynamic range /bit
Digital radiography (thorax)	1 024 x 1 024	12
	(4 096 x 4 096)	(16)
Digital angiography (DA)	1 024 x 1 024	12
	(4 096 x 4 096)	(16)
Computed tomography (CT)	512 x 512	14
Positron-emission tomography (PET)	128 x 128	16
Gamma camera	256 x 256	16
Ultrasonic imaging	512 x 512	8
Magnetic resonance imaging (MRI)	512 x 512	16

Source: J. Perry, "Performance features for a PACS display console".
Computer, vol.16, 1983, No.8, pp.51-54.

Figure II.25. Sequencing of basic image-processing operations

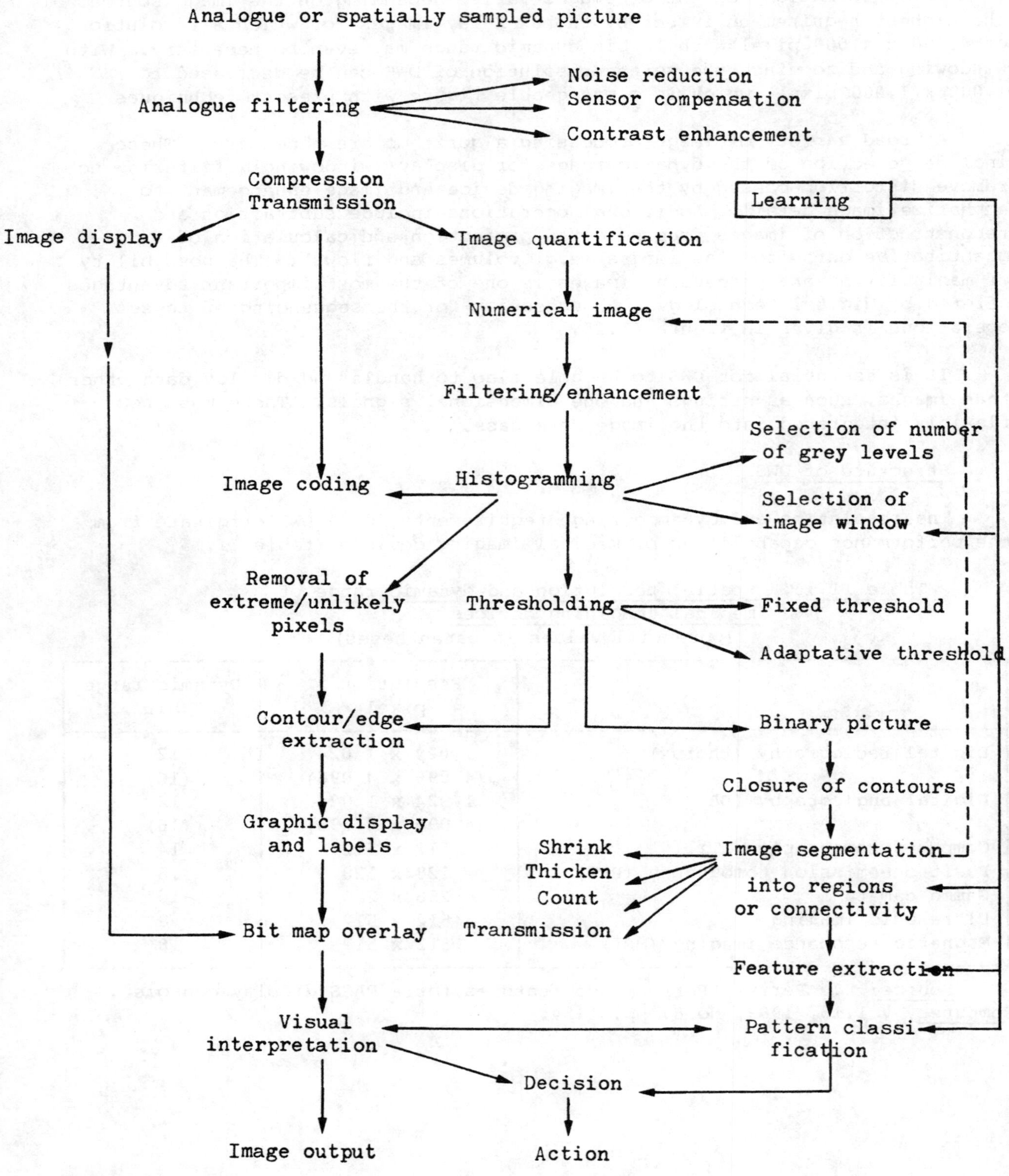

Source: Image Processing Equipment and Software. Proposal for a multi-client project. Battelle, Geneva, 1985.

The only realistic display type to fulfil these requirements is the cathode ray tube (CRT). Flat displays do not yet have the required resolution. Even with CRTs, the dynamic range is not sufficient. Instead, windowing and zooming must be used to circumvent these restrictions.

A DWS typically comprises the following components:

- Software to control and to carry out the functions specified below and software for the support of man/machine interaction;

- Several black-and-white and colour high-resolution video monitors;

- A versatile alphanumeric and command keyboard and an interactive graphic input device;

- A large enough image memory, able to support different display modes (e.g. high-resolution still images and a moving image sequence with a lower resolution);

- A flexible and fast internal bus structure to support the functions;

- Processor modules for high-speed preprocessing, compression/decompression etc., a programmable array processor for image processing and a powerful micro- or minicomputer for control of the DWS;

- A flexible interface for connecting the DWS to PACS; and

- A multiformat camera or similar copying device for hard-copy print-outs (this can also be a resource shared between many DWS).

8.5 Outlook

The PACS concept is based on three components: the image sources producing digital images, the communication network for transferring the images at a high enough speed, and the image management, processing and display system providing also the interface to the users. Of these components, the technology required for image sources mostly exists already, as evidenced by the wide variety of modalities available. However, the most important modality, the conventional X-ray, is still based on film. Communication networks today are not able fully to support the PACS environment. This is partly due to the relatively low efficiency of the networks when considering the very large volume of data involved, and partly due to the fact that international standards for network interfaces applicable to image transmission are only just emerging.

The third component, the image management processing and display system, can be (and has been) realized with present technologies. However, before they can really be utilized, their capabilities in performing image manipulations, processing and interpretation must be improved. For this, pattern recognition and artificial intelligence techniques are necessary. It is also important that the computing power of such work-stations should be high enough.

Besides intrahospital PACS, there is considerable potential for PACS in rationalizing and improving co-operation between hospitals and primary-care centres. Several products exist today that can transfer X-ray images taken in the primary-care centre to a radiologist located in a hospital. This teleradiology contact has also been tested between hospitals.

A more complete illustration of the various components that can be included in PACS is given in figure II.26.

Medical information systems (MIS) are being created both on a departmental basis as radiological information systems (RIS) and on a hospital basis as hospital information systems (HIS). These contain and communicate patient data. It is of utmost importance that PACS should be integrated to RIS and HIS for effective utilization of all patient data (see figure II.27).

The HIS of the Tokyo University Hospital includes a PACS. It covers data acquisition, a communication subsystem (LAN), a storage subsystem, a viewing station and a planning subsystem. The first phase of PACS has already been implemented and in 1986-1989 the system will be significantly enlarged (evaluation subsystem of picture quality, man-machine interfaces, on-line connection of various diagnostic units, large-scale picture data base, reporting system, etc.). The system is based on the use of FACOM computers [56] (see also chapter V - Japan).

9.   INTERNATIONAL TRADE IN ELECTROMEDICAL EQUIPMENT AND THE DIGITAL IMAGING MARKET

9.1   International trade in electromedical equipment

Electromedical equipment is identified within the United Nations Standard International Trade Classification (SITC, Rev.2) Group 774: "Electrical apparatus for medical purposes and radiological apparatus" and divided into two subgroups:

774.1   Electromedical apparatus (other than radiological apparatus); and

774.2   Apparatus based on the use of X-rays or of the radiations from radioactive substances (including radiography and radiotherapy apparatus); X-ray generators; X-ray tubes; X-ray screens; X-ray high tension generators; X-ray control panels and desks; X-ray examination or treatment tables, chairs and the like; parts, n.e.s. of and accessories for the foregoing apparatus and equipment.

The information presented in annex I is based on data from 24 major exporting (and importing) countries, as follows:

(a)   North America: Canada, United States

(b)   Europe (market-economy): Austria, Belgium-Luxembourg, Denmark, Finland, France, Federal Republic of Germany, Ireland, Italy, Netherlands, Norway, Spain, Sweden, Switzerland and the United Kingdom

Figure II.26. The scope of picture archiving and
communication systems

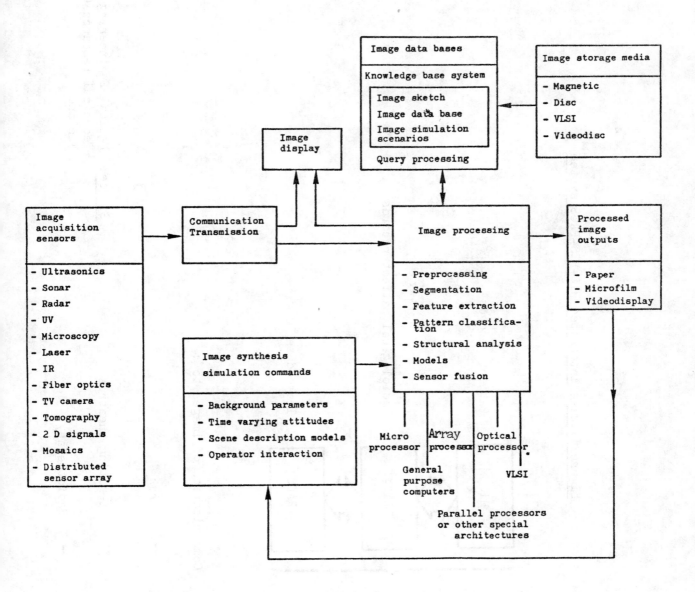

Source: As for figure II.25.

Figure II.27. Integrated HIS-RIS-PACS system

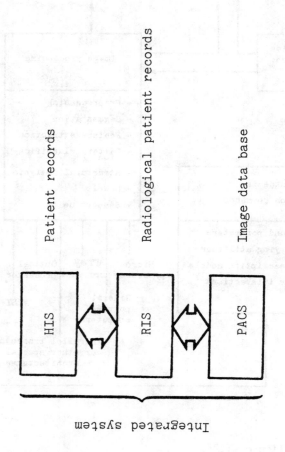

Patient records

Radiological patient records

Image data base

HIS

RIS

PACS

Integrated system

Communication of images to :

— Wards

— Operating theatres

— Radiotherapy

Source : Medical Engineering Laboratory, Technical Research Centre of Finland.

- 76 -

(c)   Europe (centrally-planned): Czechoslovakia, Poland

(d)   Asia: Hong Kong, Israel, Japan, Republic of Korea and Singapore

(e)   Oceania: Australia

The selected countries export electromedical equipment for at least
$US 1 million per year.

Annex III shows the exports and imports (and trade balance) in 1978-1985
for the above-mentioned 24 selected countries which report to the
United Nations Statistics "Comtrade Database". It demonstrates the fact that
the major exporters (countries with a positive international trade balance)
are Denmark, the Federal Republic of Germany, Japan, the Netherlands, Sweden,
the United Kingdom and the United States.

Annex IV provides a comparison between the selected and other reporting
countries concerning exports and imports of electromedical equipment. It
clearly shows that the major exporters are at the same time the dominating
importers (consumers, users) of this equipment. In the absence of data on
production, it, however, indicates the present "relative isolation" of
countries which are the dominant traders in modern (and expensive) equipment
for sophisticated health care.

In any case, the overall picture is certainly biased by the fact that
many large and important countries-producers and/or users of electromedical
equipment are still not reporting to the United Nations Statistics
"Comtrade Database". This applies e.g. to Argentina, Brazil, Bulgaria, China,
the German Democratic Republic, Hungary (reporting to the United Nations data
bank at the two-digit SITC level 77 only), India, Mexico, Romania, the USSR
and Yugoslavia. In order to illustrate the trade in electromedical equipment
of these countries, available data have been used from the UN/ECE Bulletins of
Statistics on World Trade in Engineering Industries 1983 and 1984 (see
annex V).

9.2   Market projections for digital imaging equipment

It is estimated that diagnostic imaging corresponds roughly to one third
of the total world market for medical equipment (including laboratory
equipment). The diagnostic-imaging field is large and expensive, as shown in
tables II.16 and II.17. The figures represent the situation in the
United States and are estimates. As the tables show, the use of ultrasound
has recently been growing very fast. In nuclear medicine, the number of
examinations is growing at a much slower pace. For CT scanning, as already
discussed in chapter II.2, use has increased strongly. The number of
film-based X-ray examinations seems to have reached a nearly constant plateau.

Table II.16. Overview of diagnostic imaging in the
United States for 1977 and 1980

	Number of hospitals with capability	Number of procedures (millions)		Costs (millions of US dollars)	
		1977	1980	1977	1980
Diagnostic X-ray	7 000	158	171	5 300	7 600
CT scanning	1 000	1-1.4	3-4	300	875
Nuclear medicine	3 300	8.2	11.1	800	1 250
Ultrasound	All	Approximately 4		...	360

Source: Policy implications of the computed tomography (CT) scanner. An updating Office of Technology Assessment, United States Congress. OTA-BP-H-8, January 1981, p.59.

Note: Estimates are approximate, for illustration only.

Table II.17. Sales of diagnostic imaging equipment in the United States

	Sales (millions of dollars)						
	1974	1975	1976	1977	1981	1982	1983
Diagnostic X-ray	265	300	230	280	375	-	-
CT scanning	-	100	120	160	200	-	-
Nuclear medicine	40	-	-	100	-	127	-
Ultrasound	65	-	-	160	-	269	490

Source: As for table II.16.

Note: The validity of the sales figures is not known. They are undoubtedly rough. They are included here as general indicators only.

- 78 -

Growth projections for the diagnostic-imaging market are very favourable. In connection with its MRI study, OTA published, in 1984, a projection (table II.18) according to which the major growth areas are MRI, digital X-ray and ultrasound. Modalities with decreasing market shares are conventional X-ray and CT scanners. It was projected that between 1983 and 1988 the markets would double. However, in view of the recent cost-containment efforts of health care services and the developments in 1984-1986, the projection proved to be over-optimistic.

Biomedical Business International (BBI) has published world-wide sales estimates of diagnostic imaging devices for 1984 (table II.19) that seem to indicate that the OTA projection is indeed over-optimistic. The OTA study identified ultrasound as a major growth area. Other projections, however, indicate that this market is nearing saturation. MRI sales agree in both projections, but, owing to the early stage of development, major changes are still possible. The BBI projections do not differentiate between conventional and digital X-ray. Another study predicts an annual growth rate of between 10 and 15 per cent over the next few years. [57] The OTA study projected a 15 per cent growth rate.

According to table II.19 there would be major changes in the percentages of industry sales between different imaging modalities between 1983 and 1988. MRI and CT are projected to compete for the same markets as MRI, the winner. However, CT has become an established technique in diagnostic imaging and is cheaper than MRI. Also, CT is able to image bone, which MRI cannot do. For these reasons, it is felt that CT will stay and MRI will be used to complement it in larger hospitals. The change from film-based to digital X-ray is projected to take place between 1983 and 1988. However, as already discussed in chapter II.2., digital radiography is not yet sufficiently far advanced for the OTA projection to be valid.

Table II.18. Growth projections for the world-wide sales
of the diagnostic imaging industry

| Modality | 1983* | | 1988* | | 1983 to 1988 | |
	Market size (millions of US dollars)	Percentage of industry sales	Market size (millions of US dollars)	Percentage of industry sales	Overall percentage change in market size	Annual percentage change in market size
All X-ray modalities	2 900	72.5	3 500	42.7	+ 21	+ 4
Conventional X-ray	(1 300)	(32.5)	(500)	(6.1)	(− 61)	(− 17)
Digital X-ray a/	(600)	(15.0)	(2 500)	(30.5)	(+ 317)	(+ 33)
CT	(1 000)	(25.0)	(500)	(6.1)	(− 50)	(− 13)
Ultrasound	750	18.8	1 900	23.1	+ 153	+ 20
Nuclear medicine	250	6.2	300	3.7	+ 20	+ 5
NMR	100	2.5	2 500	30.5	+ 2 500	+ 90
Total	4 000	100.0	8 200	100.0	+ 105	+ 15.0

Source: Health Technology Case Study 27. Nuclear Magnetic Resonance
Imaging Technology: A Clinical, Industrial and Policy Analysis. Washington,
DC. United States Congress Office of Technology Assessment, OTA-HCS-27,
September 1984, p.58. (Original source: R.B. Emmitt, J.W. Lasersohn "Company
Report on Diasonics"; F. Eberstadt & Co. Inc., New York, 1983).

a/ Includes both digital add-on and full-systems with a digital
capability.

Table II.19.   The world market for diagnostic
                imaging equipment, 1984
                  (Millions of US dollars)

Company	X-ray a/	CT	Nuclear medicine	Ultra-sound	NMR	1984 world-wide sales
General Electric	380	210	35	20	25	670
Siemens	340	210	50	25	20	645
Philips	300	50	–	65	20	435
GEC/Picker Intl	160	80	25	20	45	330
Toshiba	180	60	10	55	12	317
Technicare (J&J)	35	110	30	45	70	290
CGR	200	40	–	10	6	256
Hitachi	80	40	–	20	8	148
Elscint	10	80	25	10	20	145
Diasonics b/	15	–	–	75	30	120
All others	450	30	65	200	15	760
TOTAL	2 150	910	240	545	271	4 116

Source: Biomedical Business International, vol.VIII, p.153.

a/ Film-based and digital.

b/ Excludes service revenues, films, chemicals, imaging kits,
accessories and sales of image-processing systems (PACS).

Table II.20 shows the evolution of the structure of DI equipment markets
in the United States; in particular, it points to the fact that the
United States domestic market in 1984 made up nearly 50 per cent of the total
world market.

Table II.20. United States domestic market for diagnostic
imaging equipment, 1976-1986
(Millions of US dollars)

Year	X-ray	CT	Nuclear medicine	Ultrasound	NMR	Total
1976	393	112	85	75	–	665
1982	949	524	164	229	9	1 875
1983	934	751	152	237	50	2 124
1984	916	595	140	247	129	2 027
1985*	836	362	136	256	260	1 850
1986*	809	270	130	266	440	1 915

Source: Diagnostic Imaging, March 1986.
(Original source: Hambrecht & Quist estimates).

These projections do not include PACS. According to Biomedical Business
International [58] the world market for PACS in 1983 was $US 90 million.
Respectively the film recorder and processor market in 1984 is estimated at
$260 million. [59] The same source indicates that this market segment will
not be markedly affected by PACS by 1988. These figures do not include X-ray
films or processor chemicals.

In conclusion, the market will be dominated within the next few years by
sales of diagnostic imaging devices, most notably by MRI. PACS will arrive
gradually towards the end of the 1980s.

9.3 State of diffusion of imaging technologies

Based on what has been described in this chapter concerning the state of
the art of DI clinically, technologically and economically, the following
conclusions can be drawn:

- DI is a highly interdisciplinary field. Its progress depends on
  developments in many areas of information technology, such as local
  area networks, communication protocols, computer technology and
  automation means, and artificial intelligence, together with pattern
  recognition;

- The technology needed for producing medical images is advancing
  rapidly, making the life cycles of products relatively short;

- The present and projected diffusion of DI components is given in
  figure II.28. The figure to some extent disagrees with the above
  consideration of MRI. It is projected that CT will be the major
  modality over MRI and that digital radiography will not be commercially
  successful until the early 1990s;

- The integration of image sources through PACS will still require some
  years. PACS will be introduced into diagnostic imaging gradually; and

- Owing to the dynamic situation, it is not clear what will be the
  consequences of DI for health care with respect to both its clinical
  applications and its socio-economic impact on health-care costs and
  staff.

Figure II.28.   State of diffusion of DI components

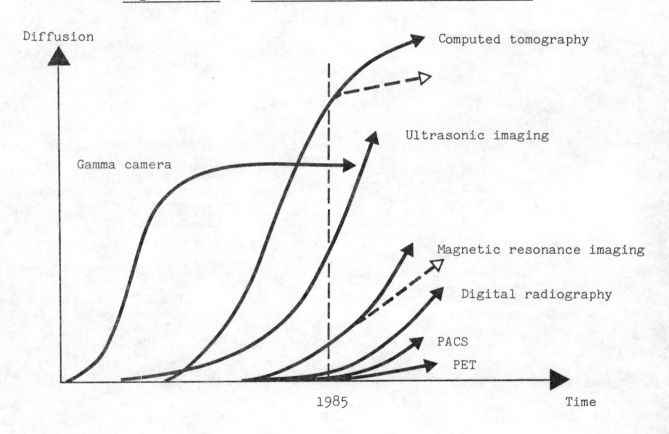

PET = positron emission tomography

PACS = picture archiving and communication system

━ ━ ━ ━► alternative projection

CHAPTER III - FACTORS INFLUENCING DIGITAL IMAGING DESIGN AND MANUFACTURE

1. EVOLUTION OF TECHNOLOGIES - MANUFACTURERS AND RESEARCH INSTITUTES

1.1 Evolution of technologies

The evolution of technologies pertinent to the DI field has been partly covered in chapter II in the presentation of the state of the art of various DI components. This was done from the application point of view. Another approach is to look at the basic technologies on which DI is based. Because of its interdisciplinary nature, DI owes its progress to many technologies, as indicated by figure III.1.

The major factors behind the present rapid development of DI can be attributed to computer technology and microelectronics. For several of the imaging modalities, discoveries in nuclear physics have provided the theoretical background for the application, such as X-rays and nuclear medicine in general, and MRI. From the point of view of computation, the newer imaging modalities are so demanding that they would not be feasible without the present capabilities of computer technology.

For the continued advancement of DI, several technologies are important (figure III.1). Digital imaging is being increasingly influenced by health economics, which provides tools for assessing the cost, efficiency and benefits of a new technology, and by the sociological sciences which provide an understanding of man/machine interaction and the motivational factors connected to it.

1.2 Manufacturers of digital imaging systems

Table III.1 lists the largest manufacturers of imaging devices in 1984. Of these, General Electric and Diasonics are United States companies, Siemens, Philips, GEC/Picker Intl and CGR are European, Toshiba and Hitachi Japanese, and Elscint Israeli. Most of these companies are multinational, however, with R and D and production spread over many countries. It should be noted that the largest companies, at least, are rather evenly distributed geographically. Of the total markets of medical imaging devices, the 10 largest companies account for 80 per cent. The rest is divided amongst several smaller companies. Table III.1 originates from the OTA study on MRI, and therefore contains only those companies that were in the MRI market at the time that study was made. Since then, several additional companies have entered the MRI market (table II.9). Most of the companies have products on several other imaging modalities as well. There are also smaller specialized companies with products on only one imaging modality. This is especially true in ultrasonics and nuclear medicine, in which the market share held by companies other than those listed in table III.1 is larger than the average share held (20 per cent).

In ultrasonics, where the share held by other companies is largest (35 per cent), companies that have been successful, besides those mentioned in table III.1, include Aloka, ATL and Hewlett-Packard.

Figure III.1. Technologies influencing the advancement of DI

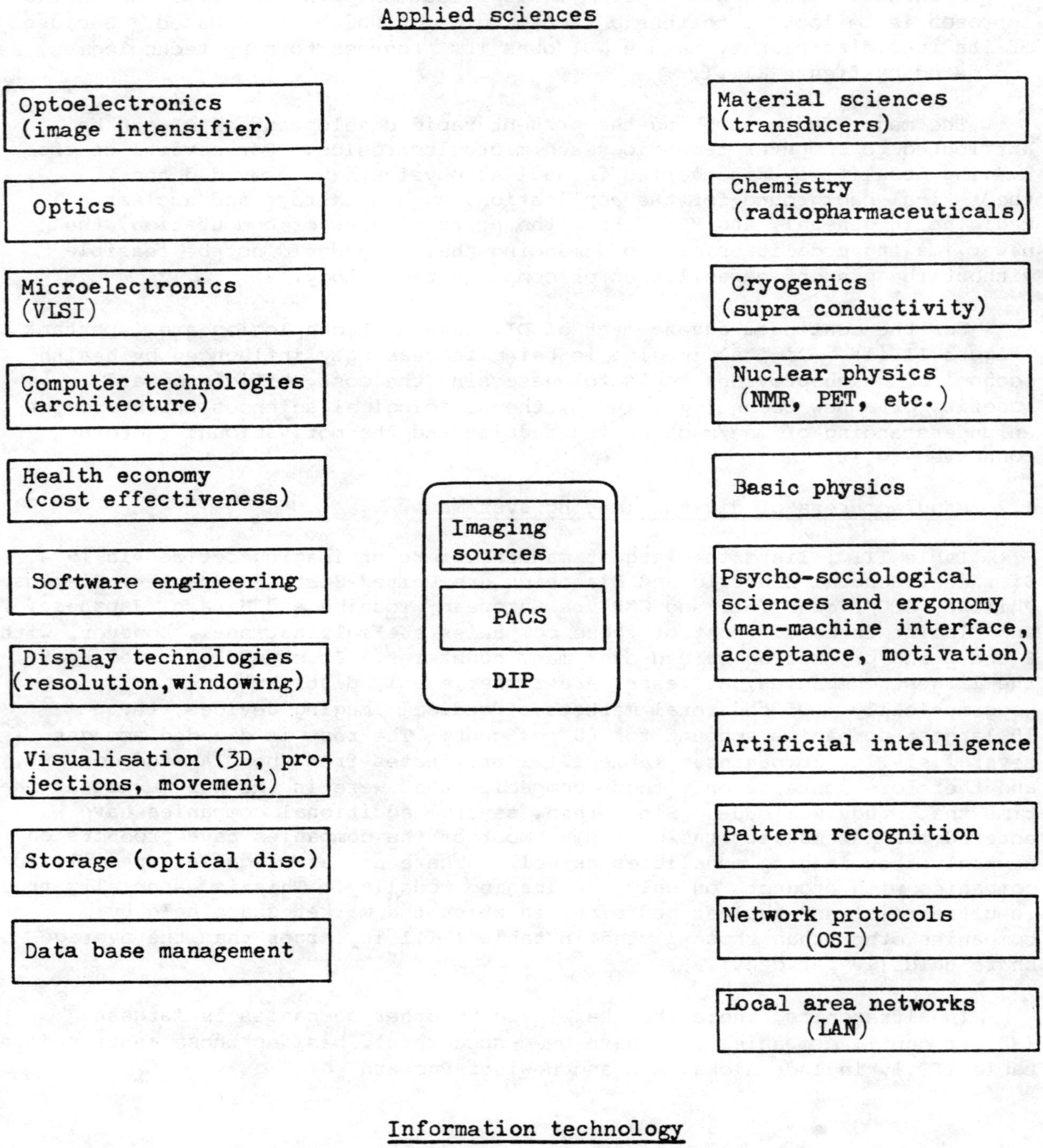

Applied sciences

Optoelectronics (image intensifier)	Material sciences (transducers)
Optics	Chemistry (radiopharmaceuticals)
Microelectronics (VLSI)	Cryogenics (supra conductivity)
Computer technologies (architecture)	Nuclear physics (NMR, PET, etc.)
Health economy (cost effectiveness)	Basic physics
Software engineering	Psycho-sociological sciences and ergonomy (man-machine interface, acceptance, motivation)
Display technologies (resolution, windowing)	
Visualisation (3D, projections, movement)	Artificial intelligence
Storage (optical disc)	Pattern recognition
Data base management	Network protocols (OSI)
	Local area networks (LAN)

Imaging sources

PACS

DIP

Information technology

Table III.1.   Non-exhaustive list of companies manufacturing medical-imaging devices

Company	CT	US	NM	DR	XR	MRI
ADAC Laboratories			X	X	X	X
CGR Medical Corp.	X	X	X	X	X	X
Diasonics Inc.		X				X
Elscint Ltd.	X	X	X	X	X	X
Fonar Corp.						X
General Electric Co.	X	X	X	X	X	X
Hitachi Ltd.	X	X	X	X	X	X
JEOL USA						X
M&D Technology Ltd.						X
Philips Medical Systems	X	X	X	X	X	X
Picker International	X	X	X	X	X	X
Shimadzu Corp.	X	X	X	X	X	X
Siemens Medical Systems	X	X	X	X	X	X
Technicare Corp.	X	X	X	X		X
Toshiba Corp.	X	X	X	X	X	X

CT = computed tomography; US = ultrasound; NM = nuclear medicine;
DR = digital radiography (mainly DA systems); XR = film-based radiography;
MRI = magnetic resonance imaging.

Source: Health Technology Case Study 27. Nuclear Magnetic Resonance Imaging Technology: A Clinical, Industrial and Policy Analysis. Washington, DC. United States Congress Office of Technology Assessment, OTA-HCS-27, September 1984, p.51 and updating by T.A. Iinuma, National Institute of Radiological Sciences, Chiba-Shi (Japan), 1986.

1.3 Research institutes

There are at present numerous companies engaged in DI research and development, most of whom are not involved with medical applications exclusively. Since the market for PACS has not yet materialized, it is impossible to establish a representative list of companies.

Contacts between companies manufacturing DI devices and research institutes are important to the industry. The companies have their own R and D laboratories that co-operate with universities, research institutes and hospitals. The larger multinational companies have contacts in many countries. It is impossible to give a complete up-to-date list of research institutes and university departments that are co-operating with the companies or otherwise contributing to the DI field. Some information in this respect is included in chapter V.

2. MANUFACTURING AND SYSTEMS INTEGRATION CONSIDERATIONS

A DI device is a typical high-technology product incorporating computer technology. To be competitive, the product must have some special features (niches). Since the hardware normally comes from a computer manufacturer, these must consist in the way the computer is programmed (software), or in the imaging-device function, or in the communication with the users or with other systems, or in all of these.

Since no internationally-accepted standards exist today for the interconnection of DI modules, manufacturers must design according to their own standards. Which of these will be successful in the long term is unclear. However, it is evident that large companies with a nearly complete spectrum of DI devices are in a better position to connect DI modules.

The OTA study on MRI identified several factors that are important for the competitive strategies of a company. First of all, the study claims that price is not believed to be the decisive factor. Instead, the ability to differentiate one's product favourably from that of a rival is important. Vertical integration may offer further advantages by raising barriers to entry for others. For product differentiation, nine non-price factors were considered important, namely, in descending order of importance: [60]

- Image quality;

- Product features and capabilities (performance);

- Product reliability;

- After-sales service;

- Delivery time;

- Long-term viability of the manufacturer;

- Guarantee against technical obsolescence;

- Collaborative research with clinical centres; and

- Training and education.

The three highest-ranking factors are directly dependent upon the R and D phase as well as several others. Regardless of the specific strategy employed by a company, it seems clear that product differentiation will be important.

Vertical integration includes corporate acquisitions and mergers, e.g. the number of companies in the CT scanner market has decreased considerably in recent years. Experiences in the CT field show that smaller companies are innovative and capable of developing high-performance products, but that they cannot market and maintain them. Instead they are taken over by other companies or choose to merge with them.

Another feature in DI is that the number of technologies involved is large. Therefore it is difficult for one company to master them all. This is especially evident in MRI. Most of the magnets used in MRI devices at present are produced by Oxford Instruments and Intermagnetics. However, most of the companies in the MRI market have plans to develop in-house capabilities to produce the magnets. The utilization of sub-contractors is very common in the DI field.

With respect to the manufacturing of DI devices, it should be remembered that the number of devices produced per company is not very large. The cost-benefits of automating the manufacturing process must be weighed against this fact. Besides computer technology, the production of imaging devices especially requires know-how in precision mechanics, although the trend is away from mechanical movements. The producers of software for DI devices face the same problems in productivity and maintenance as all software producers. Software engineering tools are still very crude. Development of software for the control functions of a DI device can generally be managed more easily than the development of software for such functions as man/machine interfaces, image manipulation and processing and image archiving.

Maintenance and repair services of a DI device are important for the company's reputation. Distributor and service networks covering the marketing area are the way to solve this. However, this can become too costly for companies with a narrow spectrum of DI products. The computer peripherals need regular servicing. This part could also be taken care of by the service network of the computer manufacturers.

3. PRODUCT DEVELOPMENT

The development of an imaging device is a highly interdisciplinary task requiring know-how in many technologies. The importance of staff expertise in R and D cannot be overemphasized. They need expertise in several fields of technology (e.g. physics, chemistry, precision mechanics, engineering and computer science). For small firms, staff recruitment may present a problem. On the other hand, many small companies are launched from university-based research giving them excellent access to R and D personnel. In those companies, however, recruitment of manufacturing and marketing know-how has been difficult.

In order to reach full production capability a corporate decision must be made to invest in R and D in a specified field to produce an experimental prototype. The prototype is tested in-house and refined according to results. Before a commercial prototype can be developed the unit must be installed somewhere outside the company for clinical testing. Clinical testing is necessary to obtain objective and critical data for further refinement of the product's performance and characteristics.

In addition, the potential customers are critical and expect the device to have been clinically validated before marketing. To overcome problems of acceptance by customers, the companies involve their customers in development and pre-marketing evaluation tasks. This can naturally cause problems in some cases with respect to impartiality, when the same persons are involved in both development and purchase. However, this should not be considered a negative factor, because close co-operation with health care is of fundamental importance for the existence of a company producing medical devices. Simultaneously, it is necessary to ensure that the products developed will be able to compete favourably with others with respect to both performance and price. It should be emphasized that hospitals also benefit from the R and D co-operation with industry through increased expertise.

4. ASSESSMENT OF TECHNICAL PERFORMANCE OF DIGITAL IMAGING

4.1 Methods

For the time being there are no international performance standards for medical-imaging devices. This is understandable in view of the rapid development in the field, which causes performance requirements to become obsolete fairly quickly. Instead, three alternatives are used:

(i)   Standards on how the manufacturer shall specify performance and other device data (disclosure standards);

(ii) Use of standard image phantoms to measure image quality; and

(iii) Assessment of the medical, economic and technical characteristics of a specific technology.

Although the requirement of disclosure of performance data might seem simple, there are problems which are responsible for it not being widely used. The main problems arise in connection with the ways in which measurements giving performance data should be made. The OTA study on MRI states for example that "the exquisite images that are helping to fuel excitement about MRI imaging have often required prolonged amounts of time that may not be practical to expect most hospitals to expend". [61] Before agreement can be reached on how measurements will be made, there will be a long lapse of time during which the technology will again have advanced to such an extent that the disclosure standard may become obsolete.

Image phantoms contain coarse and fine image details in a predetermined order. They are widely used by hospitals for all imaging modalities to check the image quality, both in acceptance testing during delivery and afterwards, during use, either periodically or in connection with fault repairs. Phantoms are available for gamma cameras, X-ray, CT, ultrasound and MRI.

The assessment of an imaging technology should also encompass its performance in relation to other competing technologies. In this respect, assessments do not give information that is specific to a certain product.

Assessment is an important methodology for health-care services to obtain objective information upon which to base decisions.   This will be further discussed in chapter IV.2 below.

Despite the existing problems, international co-operation in this field should be strengthened, in particular through such organizations as the International Electrotechnical Commission (IEC), the International Organization for Standardization (ISO) and the International Commission on Radiation Units and Measurements (ICRU).

As an example of the latest co-operation efforts, the establishment of an ISO/IEC Joint Steering Committee on Image Technology could be mentioned.   The first meeting of the Joint Steering Committee was held at Geneva in May 1986 in order to define the scope of future work based on the evaluation of existing ISO and IEC activities in related fields. [62] In particular, it was felt that, owing to the speed of developments, the field of imaging sciences and technologies (television, consumer still photography, medical imaging technology, graphic arts technology, micrographics and office image systems, including transmission methods, and image sciences common to image generation, processing and recording, including testing methods and materials and psychophysics of image interpretation) should now receive special attention. The possible modification of the current IEC and ISO organizational structures and even the creation of new more competent standardization bodies (technical committee, sub-committee) has been envisaged.

4.2 State of the art

In the present situation as described above, one must be satisfied with more or less objective comparisons of various imaging modalities. Tables III.2 and III.3 summarize the clinical, economic, technical and staff characteristics of the imaging modalities.   Table III.2 handles only technical performance and costs, whereas table III.3 also contains information on user requirements.

Table III.2.   Imaging characteristics of selected imaging modalities

Modality	SR	CR	TR	SNR	DIST	APPLIC	COST
Roentgenography	E	P	E	E	F	E	E
Fluoroscopy	F	P	E	F	F	F	F
Digital subtraction angiography	P	E	E	P	F	P	F
Computed tomography	F	E	F	P	F	F	P
Ultrasound	F	P	E	F	F	F	E
Positron-emission tomography	P	F	P	F	F	P	P
Nuclear medicine	P	P	P	P	F	F	E
Magnetic resonance imaging	P	E	P	P	F	F	P

SR = spatial resolution;   CR = contrast resolution;   TR = temporal resolution; SNR = signal-to-noise ratio;   DIST = distortion and artifacts;   APPLIC = widespread application;   COST = initial investment plus operating costs; E = excellent;   F = fair;   P = poor

Source: W.R. Hendee, "The impact of future technology on oncologic diagnosis". Oncologic imaging and diagnosis. Int. J. Rad. Oncology, Biol. and Phys., vol.12, 1983, pp.1,851-1,865.

Table III.3. Characteristics of the imaging modalities

Characteristic	Ultrasound	X-ray/CT	MRI	Nuclear medicine
Ionizing	No	Yes	No	Yes
Spatial resolution size of structures which can be resolved	Good (depends on depth of field)	Good to excellent	Excellent	Good
Tissue differentiation	Good	Fair to good	Excellent	Excellent (requires tissue or organ specific isotope)
Dynamic studies (ability to display motion)	Yes	Yes (with contrast agents) not for CT	No	Yes
Versatility (a) Areas of body	Cannot image through bone or air	All but limited by shadows and artifacts	Nearly all limitations in visualization of compact bone	All, as long as isotopes are available
(b) Planes	All (but limited depth)	Projections only, axial cross-sections for CT	All planes	Projections of organs cross-sections with emission CT
Operator skills required	Substantial	Average	Average also depends on type of magnet used	Substantial
Additional interpretation skills required (based on X-ray)	Substantial	Minimal	Very significant	Average
Installation/location Average requirements		None	Average substantial depending on type of magnet used	Very
System cost	$10,000 - $140,000	$20,000 - $1.5 mln	$0.8 mln - $1.5 mln (excluding special shielding etc.)	$75,000 - $250,000

Source: Biomedical Business International, vol.VII, 1984, p.125.

5. LEGAL AND SAFETY ASPECTS

5.1 Introduction

Legislation and safety in the DI field can be discussed separately for medical-imaging devices and PAC systems. Since imaging with X-ray uses ionizing radiation, legislation generally restricts and controls the dosages administered to patients and received by personnel working in these departments. The newer modalities - MRI and ultrasound - are especially attractive since they seem to be free of such hazards.

In most countries there is also legislation concerning the safety of electrical equipment administered by an appointed national authority. PACS and other medical information systems store patient files electronically. Data security of these files remains an open question in most countries.

More information on various national approaches towards legislation and safety standards is included in chapter V below.

5.2 Ionizing radiation

Legislation on the use of ionizing radiation does not generally specify any limits for the radiation doses produced by a medical examination. Rather, it addresses the more general aspects, and covers the appointment of a national authority to control and regulate the use of ionizing radiation in health care.

Usually, installations utilizing ionizing radiation are monitored continuously. The staff carry dosimeters and the equipment is checked periodically. The locations where ionizing radiation is produced must be specially shielded. Staff who use X-ray or nuclear imaging devices are required to be given special training in the safety aspects of ionizing radiation and in the handling of imaging devices.

Equipment faults and malfunctions often show up in images of altered quality. It is important that the operators of equipment should be able to detect these changes and take the necessary steps to correct the situation. Techniques for quality assurance in radiology have therefore been developed in many countries. In some countries (e.g. Sweden and the United States) the national authorities in this field have made their use mandatory.

5.3 Non-ionizing radiation

For the time being it is generally believed that the use of ultrasound and MRI devices is free of radiation hazards. If new evidence becomes available, this situation will be reviewed.

With diagnostic ultrasound, the power used is well below that of therapeutic ultrasound. However, the manufacturer is required to disclose information of the ultrasound energy emitted. [63] Quality-assurance procedures similar to those for radiology are available for ultrasound. For MRI devices some national guidelines have been set that deal with the static and time-varying magnetic and electromagnetic fields. [64]

5.4 Electrical safety

Digital imaging devices are electrical and thus controlled through national legislation on electricity. The requirements pertinent to imaging devices are in many countries based on IEC Publication 601-1, which gives general requirements for safety of electromedical equipment. Monitoring of compliance with these requirements ranges from mandatory pre-marketing type-tests to the use of the manufacturer's declaration of compliance with Good Manufacturing Practice (GMP) procedures.

5.5 Data security

Patient files on a computer can be accessed by anyone with sufficient know-how. The integration of medical information systems through networks makes it even more difficult to secure the files against unauthorized access. Passwords and ciphering are used to secure the data. Legislation in this field is generally lagging, owing to the rapid developments.

5.6 Performance of equipment

Medical equipment and imaging devices in particular rely more and more on information technology (i.e. both computer hardware and software) for their proper functioning. The systems function is based on a software program and and as these programs grow more complex the question of malfunctions and correctness of programs arises. It is a well known fact in the software engineering environment that it is impossible to write large and complex programs that are completely free of "bugs". This is an issue that has to be faced everywhere when developing and using software.

5.7 Product liability

It is very much in the manufacturer's interest to ensure that adequate safety and performance requirements are set for devices and that the users receive appropriate training in the use of equipment.

Malpractice suits, especially in the United States, have made manufacturers very careful about entering the field with new products before these are thoroughly tested. In other countries, while the same provisions exist, they are not as actively used by patients.

The hospital's liability also extends to the maintenance of the system, making quality assurance even more important.

CHAPTER IV - ECONOMIC AND SOCIAL CONSIDERATIONS OF DIGITAL IMAGING

1. ECONOMIC CONSIDERATIONS

A new DI device is introduced either to replace an old one or to start up a totally new activity, or a combination of both. In all cases, it will have some economic consequences. In considering the costs related to the introduction of a new technology, emphasis should be put on the overall life-cycle costs of that technology, as described below. The device can be bought or leased. In both cases the cost of utilizing the device consists of:

(i) Amortization of the purchasing investment including the current interest and inflation rates. DI technology is developing rapidly, therefore a suitable amortization period should be around five years. Film-based X-ray devices have had lives in excess of 10 years (even 20 years). If the device is leased, this cost is covered by the annual leasing payments;

(ii) Amortization of the installation costs, which in some cases may be high owing to the need to make extensive modifications to the building to accommodate the new system (e.g. for MRI the heavy permanent magnet or, in the case of resistive and superconducting magnets, the shielding). Installation costs could be included in the leasing payment. In the United States, especially, mobile imaging units are available. In these, the leasing payment also covers the van;

(iii) Operating costs, comprising salaries and fringe benefits of the personnel (physicians, X-ray technicians, secretaries, physicists, engineers etc.) and materials needed for examinations (energy, contrast agents, floppy disks, film, liquid helium and liquid nitrogen for a superconducting MRI device etc.);

(iv) Operational overheads comprising costs of administration, building etc.; and

(v) Maintenance costs, which for a DI device must be estimated at a considerably higher level than those for conventional non-digital techniques. Maintenance can be included in the leasing agreement, in which case these costs would be included in that payment.

These life-cycle costs, together with the expected years of utilization and the number of examinations per year, provide a means of calculating the break-even cost per examination. Under certain conditions, leasing may be a more economical alternative, also taking into account that the technique in that field is advancing rapidly.

Estimates of the annual costs of utilizing a certain imaging technology and the cost per examination have been made against this background. In discussing the state of the art in chapter II, reference was made to such studies for each imaging modality, when available. An approximate order for decreasing costs is (1) PET, (2) MRI, (3) CT, (4) DA, (5) digital radiography, (6) gamma camera, (7) ultrasound. It should be noted that the methodologies for using the newer modalities (such as MRI and PET) will certainly develop, resulting in more economic use of personnel time and materials. Simultaneously, the devices will improve, making additional savings in overall costs possible.

Theoretically the cost-effectiveness of various technologies can be compared in this way. However, in practice the comparison is not so easy. The costs of purchase, installation, maintenance and overheads can be obtained once it has been agreed what the amortizing time will be. The problem with operating costs is to estimate accurately how the workload of the staff of an imaging department is divided between the imaging devices. Different examinations require different amounts of personnel time. Also the costs of materials used depend on the type of examination. On the other hand, the number of examinations carried out annually depends on the capacity at which the system can operate, on the alternative technologies available and how much they are used, and on the demand for examinations.

For these reasons, the main objective of the economic evaluation would be to assess whether, on an overall basis, the investment in a digital facility represents a good use of resources. More specifically, the kinds of questions an economic evaluation should attempt to answer are:

- Does the imaging device enable the same diagnostic objectives to be met at lower cost?

- Alternatively, do overall costs increase either because costs per unit of service are higher with digital, or because the quantity of diagnostic services provided increases?

- Is any increase in costs accompanied by any demonstrable improvements in patient treatment or benefit?

The economic situation will, therefore, require a fairly broad assessment of the costs and benefits of the change to digital imaging. Furthermore, it can be seen that the economic evaluation needs to take account of the fact that a number of system variables may change following conversion to digital imaging, thereby altering the radiology department workload. A balance sheet of potential costs and benefits of a change to digital imaging is therefore set out in table IV.1. [65]

2. IMPLICATIONS FOR HEALTH CARE AND THE MEDICAL PROFESSION

2.1 Technology assessments

Experience with a number of new medical technologies, notably the CT scanner, has led several authors to propose general guidelines for the evaluation of high-technology diagnostic procedures. They all propose evaluation from a number of perspectives (technical, clinical and economic) and embody a logical sequence, beginning with studies of the technical performance of the technology to those of diagnostic accuracy and clinical effectiveness and cost-benefits of the technology. These evaluations in total are called technology assessments. The assessment of imaging technologies can be carried out at various levels, as indicated by table IV.2.

Table IV.1. Potential costs and benefits of a change
to digital imaging

Costs	Benefits
1. Additional capital costs (radiology equipment, computers, building alterations)	1. Saving in materials (e.g. film, darkroom supplies)
2. Re-training of staff	2. Saving in capital costs (e.g. darkroom and equipment, film storage space)
3. Additional radiologist time in image manipulation and interpretation	3. Saving in technician and radiologist time in image production (leading to reduction in staff or re-deployment to other useful duties)
4. Additional maintenance costs (e.g. on computers)	4. Saving in hospitalization (thereby allowing beds to be closed or re-deployed)
	5. Health benefits and higher patient utility, in terms of reduced invasiveness of procedures and fewer radiation-induced tumours
	6. Saving in patients' time costs and (possibly) lost production
plus, if the system variables change:	
5. Costs of extra diagnostic procedures resulting from the removal of the "gatekeeper" effects of risk or need for hospital admission	7. Benefits (in health terms, or in terms of resource savings) from the extra clinical procedures performed
6. Costs of extra clinical procedures arising from these extra diagnostic procedures	

Source: M.F. Drummond et al. Guidelines for the Evaluation of Digital
Diagnostic Imaging Equipment or Units, Department of Radiology, McMaster
University, Hamilton, Ontario. July 1983.

Table IV.2. Levels at which diagnostic imaging techniques
may be assessed

Level of the measurement		Typical output measures
Level 1	Image efficacy	Quality of image resolution
Level 2	Image and observer efficacy	Percentage yield of abnormal cases; percentage correct diagnoses; sensitivity; specificity
Level 3	Diagnostic efficacy	Change in order of clinicians diagnostic considerations
Level 4	Management efficacy (therapeutic decision-making)	Percentage change in therapeutic protocol Percentage change in appropriate therapy
Level 5	Patient outcome efficacy	Survival rates; percentage cures; morbidity measures; reduced worry of patient and family
Level 6	Societal efficacy (or utility)	Dollars added to GNP; age-adjusted survival rates

Source: M. Menken, et al. The Cost Effectiveness of Digital Subtraction Angiography in the Diagnosis of Cerebrovascular Disease (Health Technology Case Study 3V, OTA-HCS-34, Washington DC: United States Congress, Office of Technology Assessment, May 1985, p.19.

A guideline for assessing digital imaging technologies has recently been published. [65] Complete technology assessments as defined above are not available for DI devices. Studies have been made on digital subtraction angiography, computed tomography, magnetic resonance imaging and PACS, as mentioned in chapter II. It should be noted that, although guidelines for evaluation are necessary, they are not sufficient in that they must be accompanied by guidelines for diffusion.

2.2 Health-care services

The question of economics in relation to DI devices is connected with the way these services are made available to the patients, i.e. the extent to which they are centralized, or distributed to primary care level. Because the newer modalities are non-invasive and offer the possibility of early diagnosis in several diseases, they could be distributed. On the other hand, their annual operating costs, the fact that the utilization of their capabilities requires specialist physician attendance, and that at the primary-care level the device cannot be used at full capacity, speak against decentralization.

The most important expected benefits of the use of DI include:

- Enhanced diagnostic process (patient, radiologist);

- Improved patient care (patient, referring physician);

- Reduction in radiological retakes (patient, radiologist);

- Increased efficiency (radiologist, administration); and

- Reduced costs (administration).

In other words, the introduction of DI systems and PACS should be advantageous to all parties involved. It improves the diagnostic process, resulting in reduced costs and improved patient care. This is, of course, an idealistic vision, but it is also realistic, provided enough effort is put into the planning of the system and consideration given to the personnel and their motivation.

Traditionally, X-ray is available at primary-care level because of its relatively low cost and its clinical usefulness. The Basic Radiology System (BRS), [66] which is primarily intended for the developing countries, could be more economical at primary-care level even in the developed countries than the X-ray devices currently used. The utilization of X-ray in primary care requires a radiologist to be available (full or part-time). There have been many studies on one method used to circumvent this need, which is to transfer the X-ray images by telecommunication means to a hospital where radiologists are available (teleradiology). So far the technology for this is not cost-effective.

X-ray, CT and nuclear medicine imaging in hospitals are centralized and provide a service for the referring physicians. Ultrasound on the other hand is distributed and used by many specialists themselves and not by referral. It is reasonable to expect that this will continue. MRI will be located at the radiology department and PET with nuclear medicine. On the other hand, if disputes over the control of MRI devices develop between radiologists and other medical specialists, the market position of large X-ray manufacturing companies that have oriented their products and marketing to radiology departments might change. [67]

The full utilization of PACS requires that all patient data should be computerized and interconnected with a hospital information system.

2.3 The medical profession

The specialists who use medical imaging devices (radiologists, X-ray technicians, physicists etc.) are generally positive towards the use of technology, and participate actively in the development of DI. The new imaging modalities have so far not markedly changed the way these departments function. The general trend of emphasis on team work is evident here also. Regarding the professional structure of personnel, there is an increased demand for engineers, physicists and computer service personnel in general, while the demand for film developers, transcriptionists and archivists continues to decrease.

However, a fully digital imaging department with PACS requires a somewhat different approach on the part of the radiologists. To be acceptable, PACS should at the same time offer some additional features. There were negative experiences in the 1970s, when several companies tried to automate the process of X-ray image interpretation - report drafting and report writing using report generators. They all failed, mainly because of poor man/machine interfaces at the radiologist's end, resulting in more time spent on reading a radiograph than previously.

3.   PRECONDITIONS FOR THE USE OF DIGITAL IMAGING AND LABOUR ASPECTS

The personnel involved in the use of DI devices includes specialist physicians (radiology and nuclear medicine), X-ray technicians and nurses for patient positioning and similar tasks, film developers, secretarial assistants for word processing, assistants for image archiving and transfers, physicists, computer scientists and engineers for further method development and maintenance.

In order to use efficiently the available imaging capabilities and capacities, the staff's professional skills must be high and they must be motivated, properly organized and well managed.

When developing professional skills, special attention must be paid to the education and training of X-ray technicians and nurses (imaging technicians). This is the group that actually carries out the routine imaging operations and influences the outcome of examinations ("image quality"). Physicians only take part in the more demanding examinations. The imaging technicians need to know and understand on a minimum basic level how the imaging devices function. They must be taught methods for controlling proper functioning of the device. The ability to understand and confirm proper functioning also serves to increase staff motivation.

Quality assurance procedures need to cover the functioning of the whole department. This includes regular controls of imaging quality with phantom measurements, periodic preventive maintenance, logging of results and supervision of image quality. This can be done by the imaging technicians and the technical team.

The use of DI and PACS will probably not influence the need for physicians or imaging technicians. In a fully digital imaging department the film developers are unnecessary. The transition from film to digital will, however, be gradual. The automation of the clerical work within an imaging department (report writing, image archiving, transporting of images) will have an impact on the need for such personnel. The maintenance and upgrading of DI require physicists, computer scientists and engineers. Although maintenance can be contracted to an outside service company, the department must have adequate technical expertise of its own.

A recent PACS evaluation study suggests a comprehensive training programme (figure IV.1) that implements several training strategies, such as: [67]

- A comprehensive approach to training with explicit programmes to train personnel before, during and after installation;

- Instruction in various formats such as lecture/lab courses conducted on-site or at the vendor's facility, self-paced programmed learning featuring printed material, computer-based instruction, video tape, and on-site seminars; and

- Curriculum design that uses a building-block approach with tracks specialized for various user groups.

Figure IV.1.   Training strategy for the staff when introducing
                a fully digital imaging department

Occasional
  users

Frequent
  users

Radiology
technologists,
Nursing staff,
Physician
assistants

Radiologists

PACS staff

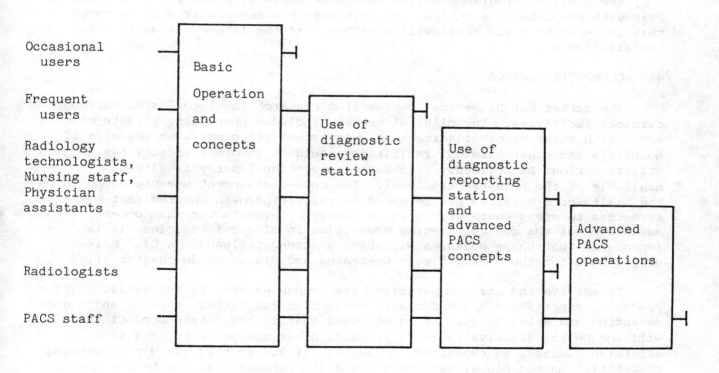

Source: Health Technology Case Study 27.   Nuclear Magnetic Resonance
          Imaging Technology: A Clinical, Industrial and Policy Analysis.
          WASHINGTON, D.C.   US Congress Office of Technology Assessment,
          OTA-HCS-27, September 1984.

There are at least six groups of users which differ on the frequency with which they use the system: [65]

- Radiologists (including radiology residents);

- Radiology technologists;

- The PACS administrators and maintainers;

- Medical staff who frequently use the services of the radiology department (orthopaedic surgeons and neurosurgeons, for example);

- Medical staff who occasionally use the services of the radiology department; and

- Nursing staff and physician assistants.

The training programme design should be aimed at providing each class of user with comprehensive skills appropriate to his needs. It must be noted that the need to train staff will continue over the life-cycle of the PACS installation.

4.   COMMERCIAL TRENDS

The market for DI devices ranges from research laboratories to various clinical facilities. The clinical segment includes hospitals, private clinics and health maintenance organizations. It is not yet clear what the size of hospitals and other clinical facilities should be in order effectively to utilize various DI devices. Film-based conventional X-ray is already available at the primary-care level. The cost-containment measures imposed on the health-care services are intended to restrict growth and redirect resources to areas where growth is necessary. Owing to the many potential advantages of the medical imaging modalities in clinical medicine, it is improbable that these measures will have a strong influence on DI. Market projections for the DI field were presented and discussed in chapter II.9.

To survive and stay competitive, the companies require innovative products, experienced R and D staff, production facilities, capital and a good marketing and sales force. It is believed that in the future product price will not be the decisive factor. Instead, other non-price factors will determine success, as explained in chapter III.2. In this rapidly developing competitive market-place, marketing and sales capabilities may be the decisive factors.

Reaching the customers in the DI field is relatively easy, as their number is rather limited. One highly cost-effective way to contact physicians is to attend and participate in commercial exhibitions organized in connection with the meetings of various medical organizations.

There have been a number of acquisitions, mergers and important trade agreements among the firms active in the DI field, mostly oriented towards product extension. A company gains entry into a related market by acquiring a firm that sells products not currently produced by the parent. Market extension mergers have also taken place. Vertical integration is common for acquiring marketing channels on foreign markets. Trade agreements are also quite frequently used to achieve this. Joint research ventures, on the other hand, are rather rare.

CHAPTER V - EXPERIENCES IN THE USE AND PRODUCTION OF DIGITAL IMAGING EQUIPMENT AND SYSTEMS

This chapter reviews national reports obtained in response to questionnaires distributed by the ECE secretariat

- In December 1985 (see annex VI); and

- In July 1986 - simplified version (see annex VII).

The second simplied questionnaire was prepared by the secretariat at the request of the second ad hoc Meeting for the study, held at Geneva from 30 June to 2 July 1986 [8] in order to encourage increased response from countries. In the absence of regular statistics in the field of digital imaging equipment and systems, the original questionnaire proved complicated and difficult to complete, even by the competent authorities of the respective countries.

The information collected from the questionnaires, although incomplete and heterogeneous, gives a unique snapshot-illustration of the ongoing process of innovation and related aspects of the introduction of DI technology in a variety of countries.

The following pages present a compilation of information received from 20 countries - Austria, Belgium, Czechoslovakia, Denmark, Finland, France, Federal Republic of Germany, Hungary, Italy, Japan, Luxembourg, Norway, Poland, Portugal, Sweden, Tunisia, Turkey, the Union of Soviet Socialist Republics, the United Kingdom and the United States. Information provided by two more countries, Bulgaria and the Netherlands (see also [82]), has been reflected in other chapters.

AUSTRIA

The number of medical imaging devices in use in Austria is shown in table V.1.

Safety legislation and standards

The Datenschutzgesetz BGBL 565/1978 has been in force since 1978.

Research and development

Government supported and university based R and D activities in the field of DI (share of public funding approx. 10 million schillings) are being carried out by the following institutions:

- Institute for Electro- and Biomedical Technology, Technical University of Graz (Professor S. Schuy); Infeldgasse 18, A-8010 Graz;

- Department of medical informatics, University Clinic of Radiology (Professor G. Gell); Auenbruggerplatz, A-8036 Graz;

- Institute for Computer Sciences in Medicine (Professor Grabner); Garnisongasse 13, A-1090 Vienna;

- Department for Remote Reconnaissance, Institute of Photogrammetry
  (Dr. F. Leberl); Rechbauerstr. 12, A-8010 Graz;

- University Clinic of Cardiology (Professor Kaindl); Spitalgasse 23,
  A-1090 Vienna; and

- Bundesinstitut für Gesundheitswesen (Dr. K. Zirm); Stubenring 6,
  A-1010 Vienna.

Table V.1.   Medical imaging devices in use in Austria (1980-1990)

Device type	Number of units in use			Number of examinations 1985
	1980	1985	1990*	
Film-based X-ray a/	3 000	3 600	4 100	12 million
Fluoroscopic X-ray	750	860	900	1.2 million
DA	14	32	65	30 000
CT scanner	20	25	55	80 000
Gamma camera	44	51	58	110 000
SPET	4	8	13	700
PET	-	-	7	-
MRI	-	-	13	-
Ultrasound	280	500	770	850 000
PACS	-	-	23	-
DWS	-	-	41	-

Source: Professor S. Schuy, Institute for Electro- and Biomedical
Technology, Technical University of Graz.

a/   Probably including dental X-ray.

BELGIUM

The Government of Belgium provided answers to both ECE questionnaires
(the first in July 1986 and its simplified updated version in
September 1986). Table V.2 shows the diffusion of various medical imaging
devices in 1985. The number of X-ray examinations in 1984 totalled some
13.13 million (provisional figure).

Table V.2.   Medical imaging devices in use in Belgium (1985-1990)

Device type	1985		Estimate 1990
	Installed	Total in use	
Film-based X-ray	20	400	replacement
Fluoroscopic X-ray	60	600	replacement
DA	20	50	replacement
CT scanner	15	50	replacement
Gamma camera	10	50	replacement
MRI	1	1	max. 10
Ultrasound	100	300	market growth

Source: Administration de l'industrie du Ministère des affaires économiques, Bruxelles.

Safety legislation and standards

There is a Royal Decree (Arrêté Royal) valid as from 28 February 1963 setting out the general regulations on the protection of the population and workers against the dangerous effects of ionizing radiation.

As regards the relevant standards in use, a Belgian standard NBN 400 exists, but it is the international standard IEC 601 on medical electrical equipment which is mainly utilized.

Policies adopted in the field of digital imaging

There is no common policy applied to the whole field, but separate approaches depending on the purchase and use of various pieces of equipment. For some of the devices, e.g. X-ray radiography, the purchase by hospitals and clinics is not restricted, whilst for others, e.g. scanners, the purchase is subject to preliminary approval of the competent public authority.

Companies active in the field

At present the only producer in Belgium is Thomson Medical Benelux, which specializes in the production of remote-control systems for radiodiagnostics and of various mobiles. It is a subsidiary of the French industrial group, Thomson-CGR. The company's turnover in the field amounted to 2,389 x 10^9 Belgian francs in 1984.

The other main suppliers of foreign-made equipment are Philips & MBLE and the Siemens group. The total turnover of Thomson, Philips and Siemens reached BF 31,073 x 10^9 in 1984.

Research and development

The R and D expenditures of Thomson Medical Benelux accounted for some 6 per cent of turnover corresponding to production activities. The company closely co-operates with most of the Belgian universities. Certain R and D projects receive interest-free advances from Government and public sources which are reimbursed by income from the sale of prototypes.

CZECHOSLOVAKIA

The number of medical imaging devices in use in Czechoslovakia is shown in table V.3.

Table V.3. Medical imaging devices in use in Czechoslovakia (1980-1990)

Device type	1980		1985		1990 *		Number of examinations 1985
	Inst-alled	Total in use	Inst-alled	Total in use	Inst-alled	Total in use	
Film-based X-ray	25	320	40	360	60	410	12.4 million
Fluoroscopic X-ray	25	180	20	190	20	190	10.2 million
Digital X-ray	-	-	...	2	...	...	...
DA	-	-	...	2	...	12	7 500
CT scanner	...	...	...	8	...	25	31 500
Gamma camera	-	3	1	5	2	10	...
PET	-	-	-	-	-	1	-
MRI	-	-	1	1	1	6	...
Ultrasound	1	3	5	20	10	40	...
PACS	-	-	-	-	...	5	-
DWS	-	-	-	-	...	5	-

Source: Dr. L. Ambroz, VUZT-CHIRANA Research Institute for Medical Engineering, Brno.

Safety legislation and standards

National standards concerning physiological safety (feasible irradiation) and respecting internationally adopted measures (e.g. WHO) are included in the CSN 40 class of standards. Regarding electrical safety, the CSN 4800 standard "Electrical medical devices" has been issued.

Technology assessment

As from 1984, systematic efforts have been made in the techno-economic assessment, including cost-effectiveness, of the introduction of digital imaging devices into medical practice. The Conference "Digital Image Processing '85" was held in Prague in 1985. Several publications on various aspects of DI technology have been issued by the VUZT-CHIRANA Research Institute for Medical Engineering (Brno), the TESLA-VUST Research Institute for Communication Technology (Prague) and the electrotechnical faculty of the Brno Technical University (VUT-FET) (see [68-71]).

Companies active in the field

The main producer of medical devices is the CHIRANA Company with headquarters at Stara Tura (Western Slovakia). It consists of seven manufacturing enterprises in various parts of Czechoslovakia, the VUZT research institute at Brno and the UZO specialized trade organization at Piestany (the watering-place where the ECE Seminar "Automation Means in Preventive Medicine '87" will be held from 28 September to 2 October 1987). [9] CHIRANA produces and supplies a wide range of surgical instruments, electronic equipment for diagnosis, X-ray technology, various therapeutic devices, sterilizers, etc. The share of DI technology is some 5 per cent of total turnover. Research expenditure amounts to 8-10 per cent of the company's profit and, in addition, several selected research programmes have received important Government funding. CHIRANA also has close R and D co-operation with leading national institutions such as the IKEM-Institute of Clinical and Experimental Medicine in Prague and the Centre for Electro-Physiological Research of the Slovak Academy of Sciences at Bratislava, as well as with the specialized departments of technical universities at Bratislava, Brno, Kosice, etc.

The largest Czechoslovak producer of measuring and laboratory devices is the TESLA (Merici a laboratorni technika) Company with headquarters at Brno and five manufacturing plants spread over the country. TESLA products in this field are exclusively based on the use of electronics (preferably applying TESLA microelectronic components and parts manufactured by another TESLA company at Roznov pod Radhostem). The TESLA R and D budget in medical applications receives significant support from centralized Government sources.

All CHIRANA and TESLA establishments report to and their activities are co-ordinated by the Federal Ministry of the Electrotechnical Industry in Prague (FMEP).

Research and development

The annual research and development expenditures of these companies are broken down as follows: basic research approximately 3.5 million Czechoslovak koruny, applied research 6 million and development 3.2 million. The major research projects include:

- Conversion of X-ray and ultrasound signals into digital form for processing and recording (co-ordinator Department of Automation and Measuring Techniques, Electrotechnical Faculty, VUT-Technical University of Brno);

- Computer means for digital image processing (Department of Theoretical Cybernetics, VSSE-Technical University of Pilsen, and Electrotechnical Faculty of the CVUT-Technical University in Prague);

- Development of nuclear magnetic resonance devices, including research in digital signal processing chains (Institute of the Theory of Measurement and Measuring Technology, Slovak Academy of Sciences, Bratislava).

International co-operation

As an example of successful international co-operation in the field of digital image processing, the bilateral agreement on scientific and technological co-operation between the USSR Ministry of Instrument Making, Automation Means and Control Systems (MINPRIBOR) and the Czechoslovak Ministry of the Electrotechnical Industry (FMEP) could be mentioned. The CHIRANA Works are in particular responsible for research and development activities in the field of X-ray image intensifiers.

DENMARK

In their answer to the ECE questionnaire, the competent authorities of Denmark provided information on digital imaging devices in use, as shown in table V.4.

Table V.4. Medical imaging devices in use in Denmark (1980-1990)

Device type	Number of units in use		
	1980	1985	1990*
Fluoroscopic X-ray	3	10	20
DA	-	5	20
CT scanner	5	19	25
Gamma camera	20	42	60
SPET	-	3	6
PET	-	-	1
MRI	-	1	3
Ultrasound	20	100	210
PACS	-	-	2
DWS	-	-	2

Source: National Agency of Technology, Ministry of Industry, Copenhagen.

FINLAND

The Government of Finland, in its answer to the simplified questionnaire, provided figures on the number of medical imaging devices in use, as shown in table V.5.

Table V.5.   Medical imaging devices in use in Finland (1980-1990)

Device type	Total number of units in use			Number of examinations 1985
	1980	1985	1990*	
Film-based X-ray a/	...	2 100	...	)
				) 4.5 million
Fluoroscopic X-ray	...	620	...	)
				)
DA	...	5	...	1 700
CT scanner	...	26	...	54 000
Gamma camera	)	35	39	)
	) 39			) 90 000
SPET	)	14	26	)
	)			)
MRI	...	3	...	...
Ultrasound	100	...	...	400 000

Source: Dr. S. Rannikko, Centre for Radiation Safety in Finland.

a/   Probably including dental X-ray.

Companies active in the field

The three main domestic producers and suppliers of medical image technology in Finland are:

- Instrumentarium/Palomex (X-ray equipment, low field MRI);

- Soredex (X-ray equipment);   and

- Nokia/Salora Company (image work-stations, image memories for DA).

FRANCE

Two French organizations contributed to the present study:

- The Regional Hospital of Nantes, introducing the DIMI project
  (Y. Bizais, Centre Hospitalier Régional, Hôpital G. & R. Laennec,
  44035 Nantes Cédex); [72]   and

- The Rennes University Hospital, implementing the SIRENE project, in co-operation with CCETT - Centre commun d'études de Télédiffusion et Télécommunications (R. Renoulin, CCETT, rue de Clos Courtel, BP 59, 35510 Cesson-Sévigné). [73]

Both, the DIMI and the SIRENE projects have received official Government support aimed at encouraging R and D activities in DI and PACS in France, based on the experience received from pilot installations at Nantes and Rennes.

At present, there are some 5,000 imaging sites in France, both public and private. They include 668 public hospitals and 860 private clinics and hospitals. In 1982, the whole field of radiology employed some 46,000 persons, with an average of three doctors and six paramedical employees per site. Radiological activities represented 2.1 per cent of total health-care expenses in 1984 (some 4 billion French francs). The total health care expenses as a share of GNP increased from 4.3 per cent in 1960 to 9.3 per cent in 1983.

The main producer and supplier of DI equipment in France is the CGR (Compagnie Générale de Radiologie), a subsidiary of Thomson. CGR at present employs some 5,000 people and about 70 per cent of the production is exported (e.g. in 1985 CGR sales were greater in the United States than in France). [74]

Additional information concerning the French national programme on the introduction of scanning and NMR equipment in 1987 was received from the WHO Regional Office in January 1987.

By the end of 1986, 29 NMR devices were authorized for delivery and use (21 in public hospital centres, 8 in private establishments). Of those NMR devices, 13 were in full-time operation in October 1986. Regarding the distribution by region, it is intended to install one NMR device for a maximum of 2.5 million inhabitants.

As concerns the introduction of CT scanners, 266 devices were authorized for delivery and use by the end of 1986 (182 in public hospitals and 84 in private establishments). More than 200 CT scanners were in full-time operation in October 1986. The indicator of needs has been set to one scanner per 170-330,000 inhabitants.

The French Ministry of Social Affairs and Employment, Ministry of Health and Family and the Directorate of Hospitals have launched a national programme (including several inquiries) aimed at controlling the diffusion of expensive CT and NMR equipment and its utilization and the access to it by various geographical areas.

An analysis of the frenquency of use of CT and NMR devices installed in 1985 showed that the average number of examinations per device varied from 3,600 to 8,000 per year (extremum values from 1,700 to 10,000 per year), depending on the type of device and the category of the establishment.

FEDERAL REPUBLIC OF GERMANY

The number of medical imaging devices in use in the Federal Republic of Germany is presented in table V.6.

Table V.6.   Medical imaging devices in use in the Federal
Republic of Germany (1980-1990)

Device type	Number of units in use			Number of examinations 1985
	1980	1985	1990*	
Digital X-ray	50	150	500	...
Other X-ray a/	27 000	30 000	32 000	40 million
DA	10	200	350	200 000
CT scanner	250	380	400	1.2 million
Gamma camera	600	800	900	1 million
PET	1	6	12	18 000
MRI	-	35	120	80 000
Ultrasound	10 000	15 000	25 000	15 million
PACS	-	1	50	...
DWS	-	5	400	...

Source: Professor H. Lemke, Institute for Technical Informatics, Technical University of Berlin.

a/   Probably including dental X-ray.

Table V.7 provides an example of the structure of DI examinations by different imaging modalities at the Radiology Department of the University Hospital of Tübingen, where in 1983 the data content amounted to nearly 70 G Bytes. Simultaneously more than 108,000 film-based examinations were made. The digital examinations represent 20 per cent of the total load of the Radiology Department. Estimating the amount of data needed to represent these films digitally, one arrives at a total figure of more than 7,000 GBytes. [75]

Table V.7. Number of digital imaging examinations at
Tübingen (1983)

Imaging modality	Number of examinations	Data content (G Bytes)
CT (body)	4 817	37.86
CT (head)	8 382	8.30
DA	494	6.47
Ultrasound	7 309	15.35
Nuclear imaging	6 664	1.20
Total	27 666	69.18

Source: W. Bautz and J. Kolbe, Is PACS feasible for a Major Department
of Radiology. Digit. Bilddiagn. 6(1986)43-48. In German.

As regards the outlook, a forecast published by Prognos for the average
size hospital in the Federal Republic of Germany estimates that, in 1990,
50 per cent of the images will be digital, whereas the percentage in 1985 was
20 per cent (table V.8). The table also shows the imaging sources. Digital
radiography will be available at the end of the 1980s. By 1995, most of the
images will be produced digitally. The dominant image source will continue to
be the conventional X-ray. MRI's share of the images will increase rapidly,
partly at the expense of CT.

Table V.8. Estimated growth of the share of DI examinations in
the Federal Republic of Germany (1985-1990)
(Percentage)

Imaging modality	1985	1990 *	1995 *
X-ray computer tomography	6	5	4
Digital subtraction radiography	2	3	3
Ultrasound	5	6	7
Nuclear medicine	7	6	6
Magnetic resonance imaging	-	5	10
Digital radiography	-	25	50
Share of DI in total examinations	20	50	80

Source: "Computer Assisted Radiology", study by PROGNOS, Basel
(published with permission of PROGNOS).

The competent Hungarian authorities, in reply to the ECE questionnaire, provided the information which follows. The number of DI devices in use in Hungary is shown in table V.9.

Table V.9. Medical imaging devices in use in Hungary (1980-1990)

Device type	1980		1985		1990*		Number of examinations 1985
	Inst-alled	Total in use	Inst-alled	Total in use	Inst-alled	Total in use	
Film-based X-ray	13	620	5	620	50	620	9.845 million
Fluoroscopic X-ray	26	1 230	20	1 250	70	1 250	1.073 million
Digital X-ray	-	-	-	-	5	10	-
DA	-	-	1	1	5	10	1 750
CT scanner	-	2	-	3	2	10	8 290
Gamma camera	5	11	4	32	5	60	141 300
SPET	-	-	-	-	5	10	-
PET	-	-	-	-	-	1	-
MRI	-	-	-	-	2	5	-
Ultrasound	8	12	12	68	10	140	262 000
PACS	-	-	-	-	-	1	-

Source: Dr. P. Vittay, Postgraduate Medical School, Budapest.

Companies active in the field

The two main producers and suppliers of digital imaging equipment in Hungary are the Medicor Company and the Gamma Müvek Company.

Medicor is a public enterprise with 35 years' experience in the field of X-ray, and six years' experience in DI, manufacturing a wide range of biomedical products such as disposable needles, laboratory devices, electro-medical devices and X-ray equipment. Its R and D investment amounts to 5 per cent of its total turnover.

Gamma Müvek was established some 65 years ago. It specializes in nuclear medicine devices, geophysical equipment and process control instruments. The company has been making complete laboratories for nuclear medicine for

25 years and image processing equipment for nuclear medicine for 10 years. It has its own development capacity, and has connections with other development institutes. Its R and D investment is about 11 per cent of its total turnover.

Table V.10 provides basic information on the production and international trade of Medicor and Gamma Müvek.

Table V.10. Hungarian companies active in digital imaging

Company	Main products in DI	Turnover (million US dollars) in DI	Total	Markets Home/Export (per cent/per cent)	Recipient countries
Medicor	CT scanners	4.0		10/90	USSR, German Dem. Rep., Peru, Cyprus, China, Turkey, Brazil, Iran, Mozambique
	Ultrasound devices	1.5		80/20	
	Diagnostic workstations	0.1		50/50	
	Total Medicor	5.6	100		
Gamma Müvek	Gamma cameras (from 1978)	25.0		15/85	Centrally-planned countries of eastern Europe, Turkey, African countries, Brazil
	Image processing equipment for gamma-cameras (from 1976)	27.0		15/85	
	Ultrasono-graphy (from 1985)	0.5		100/0	

Source: T. Vadas, Ministry of Industry (IPARI), Budapest.

Research and development

Government support amounting to some $US 0.25 million was allocated for R and D in the field of DI in Hungary in the period 1981-1985.

- 114 -

ITALY

The Government of Italy, in answer to the simplified questionnaire, provided figures on the number of DI devices in medical use, as shown in table V.11.

Table V.11. Medical imaging devices in use in Italy (1980-1990)

Device type	Number of units in use			Number of examinations 1985
	1980	1985	1990*	
X-ray all types a/	8 000	8 000	8 800	34 million
DA	140	230	250	460 000
CT scanner	80	250	320	900 000
Gamma camera	250	350	390	1 million
SPET	2	50	130	15 000
PET	-	1	6	...
MRI	-	6	40	10 000
Ultrasound	380	2 800	3 500	3.5 million
PACS	-	4	...	...
DWS	-	2	...	...

Source: Ministry of Industry, Rome.

a/ Probably including dental X-ray.

According to information provided by the WHO Regional Office for Europe, the DI equipment market in Italy is dominated by foreign manufacturers (CGR, Diasonics, Elscint, General Electric, Philips and Siemens) with shares from 85 to 100 per cent. Italian producers have a 10 per cent market share in digital radiology (Gilardoni), 10 per cent in NMR (Ansaldo) and 15 per cent in Gamma cameras (Selo). CT scanners are exclusively imported.

JAPAN

Several Japanese organizations contributed to the present study:

- The Faculty of Medicine, University of Tokyo (Professor M. Saito and Professor M. Iio);

- The Institute of Industrial Science, University of Tokyo (Professor M. Onoe);

- The Section of Medical Physics and Engineering, Division of Clinical
  Research, National Institute of Radiological Sciences, Chiba-shi
  (Dr. T.A. Iinuma);

- Systems and Software Department, Medical Systems Division, Toshiba
  Corporation, Tochigi-ken (Dr. K. Kita); and

- Department of Radiology, National Defense Medical College,
  Tokorozawa-shi (Professor E. Takenaka).

Their contributions and comments on the draft study have already been included
in other relevant chapters. In the absence of official figures for the total
number of DI devices in use in Japan, the level of use of DI equipment might
be illustrated by an example of the current installations at the University of
Tokyo:

- 1 MRI system (1.5 T);
- 1 DA system;
- 5 CT scanners;
- 2 digital radiography systems (Fuji, Toshiba);
- 5 gamma cameras (2 SPECT); and
- 1 PACS.

Recent developments in DI equipment and systems were discussed at the
Fifth Symposium on Medical Imaging Technology (held in conjunction with the
Third International Symposium on PACS and PHD) in Tokyo from 9 to
12 July 1986. Both symposia were co-sponsored by the Japan Society of PACS
(JAPACS).

The Japan Association for the Advancement of Medical Equipment (JAAME)
was established in 1985 with the following objectives and activities:

The Association is intended for the research and development of medical
equipment and the investigation and study of its production, export and
import, distribution, layout and use. At the same time, it aims at
promoting and encouraging the adequate extension and improvement of
medical equipment and the sound development of the medical equipment
industry with a view to contributing to the promotion of the health of
the people and the advancement and improvement of medical science.

JAAME engages in the following activities:

- Research and development of, and experiments concerning medical
  equipment and the provision of subsidies for the foregoing.

- Investigation and study, and collection and offer of information
  concerning research and development, production, export and import,
  distribution, layout and use of medical equipment.

- Guidance and other necessary technical support to medical organs and
  medical equipment enterprises related to research and development, etc.

- Training of medical equipment operators and engineers.

- Issuing of the required publications and sponsoring of lecture meetings.

- Co-ordination and co-operation with overseas and Japanese agencies and organizations relating to medical equipment.

- Any other activities required to achieve the above objectives.

These operations are carried out through close co-operation with the health and welfare administration and with the participation of medical equipment enterprises, medical personnel and medical and engineering researchers.

In 1985, JAAME started work on two "entrusted" projects (medical equipment data bank, study on application fields) and four more general projects, including an overseas co-operation project.

LUXEMBOURG

Medical imaging devices in use

According to the information provided by the competent authorities of Luxembourg, the following DI devices were in use in 1985:

- Some 300 film-based and fluoroscopic X-ray units;
- 4 digital X-ray units;
- 4 DA devices;
- 2 computer tomographs;
- 3 gamma cameras;
- 1 single photon-emission tomograph; and
- Some 15 ultrasound devices.

Legislation and safety standards

Hospitals wishing to purchase medical or medico-technical equipment costing more than 1,553,000 Luxembourg francs (including VAT) must obtain prior authorization from the Minister of Health (Law of 29 August 1976 on the planning and organization of hospitals). Authorization is granted when the equipment is deemed necessary for public health, as covered by regulation of the Grand Duchy of Luxembourg (National Hospital Plan of 30 March 1982).

Equipment for use in doctors' consulting rooms is controlled by a Government regulation (Law of 29 April 1983) covering the medical, dental and veterinary professions.

Electric equipment used in human medicine must comply with the technical specifications of the Government regulation of 8 August 1985 covering electric apparatus for use in human and veterinary medicine.

In furtherance of the law of 10 August 1983 concerning the medical use of ionizing radiation, a regulation at present under preparation will determine the minimum obligatory characteristics and performances of radiological equipment, according to the category of examinations for which it is intended.

NORWAY

The Directorate of Health, in its answer to the simplified questionnaire (September 1986), provided information on the diffusion of digital imaging devices in Norway (see table V.12).

In the absence of a DI industry in Norway, the country at present depends on imports. Co-operation in the field of research and development is established, particularly with other Nordic countries.

Table V.12. Medical imaging devices in use in Norway (1980-1990)

Device type	Total number in use			Number of examinations 1985
	1980	1985	1990*	
Film-based X-ray a/	1 328	1 400	1 480	)
Fluoroscopic X-ray	1 100	1 120	1 150	)
DA	-	6	30	) 2.6 million
CT scanner	12	38	50	)
Gamma camera	23	30	35	) 60 000
SPET	-	1	3	)
MRI	-	-	10	-
Ultrasound	130	175	250	...
PACS	-	-	5	-

Source: Idunn Eidheim, Environmental Health Department, Directorate of Health, Oslo.

a/ Probably including dental X-ray.

POLAND

Information on the number of medical imaging devices in use was provided by the Polish authorities in January 1987.

The number of film-based X-ray devices will increase from 3,800 units in 1985 to 4,200 units in 1990, fluoroscopic X-ray devices from 1,200 to 1,800 units, DA units from 5 to 15 units, CT scanners from 14 to 20 units, gamma cameras also from 14 to 20 units and ultrasound imaging devices from 240 to 600 units.

Regarding DI devices not as yet in use in 1985, it is estimated that, by 1990, the following will be implemented: 2-3 SPET units; 2-3 PET units; 2-5 NMR systems; and 1-2 PACS.

The main manufacturers of X-ray technology (e.g. Farum, Warszawa) concentrate on the domestic supply of various devices, such as fluoroscopic X-ray devices equipped with TV monitors (annual production 80 units).

PORTUGAL

The number of medical imaging devices in use in Portugal is presented in table V.13.

In the absence of a domestic DI industry, the country at present is fully dependent upon imports.

Safety regulations and standards in the field of DI are covered by Government decrees No. 44060 of 25 November 1961 and No. 45 of 13 July 1963.

Table V.13. Medical imaging devices in use in Portugal (1980-1990)

Device type	1980		1985		Total in use 1990*
	Installed	Total in use	Installed	Total in use	
Film-based X-ray	36	747	37	814	880
Fluoroscopic X-ray	3	32	10	111	160
Digital X-ray	-	-	4	4	30
DA	-	-	5	5	20
CT scanner	2	2	11	22	30
Gamma camera	-	3	2	15	20
SPET	-	1	1	6	10
PET	-	1	-	1	5
MRI	-	-	-	-	5
Ultrasound	3	3	93	209	500
PACS	-	-	-	-	5
DWS	-	-	-	-	10

Source: Permanent Mission of Portugal to the United Nations Office at Geneva.

SWEDEN

Sweden is one of the countries which has strongly supported the work on the present study. Thus, several parts of its national contribution have already been included in previous chapters. Table V.14 provides information on medical imaging devices in use.

Safety legislation and standards

No special safety regulations have been developed dealing specifically with digital imaging in health care. Traditionally, Sweden prefers to adopt internationally accepted standards, e.g. IEC 601.1.

Table V.14. Medical imaging devices in use in Sweden (1980-1990)

Device type	Total number in use			Number of examinations 1985
	1980	1985	1990*	
Film-based X-ray	800	800	...	4 million
Fluoroscopic X-ray	170	180	170	...
DA	-	8	...	3 000
CT scanner	18	45	...	80 000
Gamma camera	65	90	...	80 000
SPET	5	25	...	...
PET	1	2	2	450
MRI	0	2	8	1 500
Ultrasound	100	250	300	250 000
PACS	-	-	3	-
DWS	-	-	10	-

Source: Silas Olsson, Swedish Planning and Rationalization Institute of Health and Social Services (SPRI), Stockholm.

Purchasing policy and digital imaging assessment

The Federation of Swedish County Councils has recommended that the purchase of MRI equipment should be restricted to the regional hospitals (i.e. university hospitals). The Swedish Planning and Rationalization Institute of Health and Social Services (SPRI) has made evaluations of the use of computerized tomography (CT), digital angiography (DA) and magnetic resonance imaging (MRI) (see [23, 25, 50]).

Companies active in the field

All the major companies on the Swedish DI market (Siemens, Philips, CGR, GE) also have manufacturing facilities abroad.

There are two big international companies dominating the market in Sweden - Siemens and Philips. Siemens has a good stake in the production of medical equipment in Sweden, but not particularly in the DI sector. Philips has a marginal production of medical equipment in Sweden, but no DI products.

Research and development

The Swedish National Board for Technical Development (STU) supports research and development projects in the DI sector. A foundation owned jointly by STU and the Federation of Swedish County Councils also supports DI projects.

STU annually spends about 1-2 million Swedish kronor in the DI sector.

International co-operation

There are several international R and D co-operation projects in the DI field e.g. university hospitals which co-operate with companies on medical application software development.

Another project, on a Nordic basis, is the CART (Computer-Aided Radiotheraphy) project (see also figure II.13).

TUNISIA

Following the active interest of Tunisia in ECE activities in the field of biomedical engineering and the working contacts established during the ECE Seminar on Innovation in Biomedical Equipment (Budapest, Hungary, May 1983), the competent authorities of that country were invited to contribute to the present study. In answer to the ECE questionnaire, the Ministry of Public Health provided valuable information in the form of an analytical study on the present state of (first half of 1986) and prospects in radiology, based on a representative national inquiry. Relevant parts of the contribution are presented below and may well serve as an illustration of an effective approach towards the assessment of medical technology in a non-ECE country.

There are at present 67 Tunisian radiologists (most of them educated in France) and 25 foreign radiologists employed by university-based hospitals (some 60 per cent) and other clinics and public establishments (some 20 per cent), or working privately. Their distribution by seven main regions is shown in table V.15.

The number of radiologists per 100,000 inhabitants at the beginning of 1986 (1.26) represents a significant improvement in comparison with the situation in 1975 (approx. 0.2).

Table V.15 also shows that a large number of specialized physicians practise in the capital (Tunis-district) and the Centre-East region (Nabeul, Sfax). Another interesting result of the inquiry showed that 68.3 per cent of radiologists are under 40 and 93.7 per cent under 50 years of age.

As regards the number of devices in use, the analysis, logically, showed a similar uneven geographic distribution (see table V.16). Radiotherapy and nuclear medicine facilities are available only in the capital, DA is available in four university centres only (Tunis, Sousse, Monastir, Sfax), etc.

Table V.15. Geographic distribution of radiology
services in Tunisia (1986)

Region	Total population	Number of radiologists	Number of radiologists per 100 000 inhabitants
Tunis-district	1 394 749	44	3.16
North-East	974 818	7	0.72
North-West	1 103 845	6	0.55
Central-East	1 449 396	23	1.59
Central-West	1 008 094	4	0.40
South-East	636 234	3	0.47
South-West	399 037	1	0.25
Non-allocated (retirement, etc.)	.	4	.
Total	6 966 173	92	1.26

Source: Ministry of Public Health, Tunis.

Table V.16 Number of selected medical devices in use in Tunisia (1986)

Regions	Share of total population (percentage)	Conventional radioscopy			Fixed radiography			Mobile radiography			TV mobile radioscopy			Radio-photography			Dental X-ray			Echography		
		PB	PR	T	PB	PR	T	PB	PR	T	PB	PR	T	PB	PR	T	PB	PR	T	PB	PR	T
Tunis - district	20.0	19	75	94	61	28	89	45	4	49	8	3	11	7	1	8	15	243	258	20	23	43
North-East	14.0	16	54	70	14	6	20	4	-	4	-	-	-	1	-	1	10	30	40	2	2	4
North-West	15.9	16	27	43	20	-	20	3	-	3	1	-	1	3	-	3	8	15	23	1	-	1
Central-East	20.8	16	70	86	39	14	53	29	4	33	8	4	12	3	-	3	20	67	87	9	4	13
Central-West	14.5	13	20	33	9	-	9	4	-	4	-	-	-	1	-	1	7	4	11	-	-	-
South-East	9.1	4	24	28	10	1	11	12	2	14	2	-	2	2	-	2	4	15	19	-	-	-
South-West	5.7	6	9	15	10	-	10	6	-	6	1	-	1	1	-	1	3	10	13	-	-	-
Total	100.0	90	279	369	163	49	212	103	10	113	20	7	27	18	1	19	67	384	451	32	29	61

Source: As for table V.15.
(PB = public, PR = private, T = total)

- 123 -

Another important indicator of the health-care level is the consumption of radiological films per capita, as presented in table V.17. Whilst it showed a significant increase during the period 1976-1985, it was still well below the level reached in 1981 in such countries as the Federal Republic of Germany (0.18 m^2 per capita), France (0.23), Spain (0.15), but higher than that of Egypt (0.02).

Table V.17. Consumption of radiological films
in Tunisia (1976-1985)

Year	Film consumption in m^2	Consumption in m^2 per capita
1976	111 478	0.019
1979	170 272	0.027
1982	247 535	0.037
1985	279 657	0.039

Source: As for table V.15.

Legislation and safety standards

The legislation system in the field of ionizating radiation has been well established, in co-operation with the International Atomic Energy Agency (IAEA) and the World Health Organization (WHO). The law of 18 June 1981 provides basic regulations concerning the purchase, installation and use of medical equipment producing ionizing radiation.

Outlook

Already in the course of 1986, the decision was taken to enrich the quantity and quality of health-care services by the purchase of some 50 simple radiological systems for use in undeveloped rural areas, as well as 15 radiological systems with remote control, 20-25 echography devices and 3 CT scanners (for entire body examinations) to be installed in the public sector (Tunis, Monastir, Sfax). The trend towards the increased use of digital imaging equipment, will be accompanied by:

- Increased education and training efforts in both public and private sectors, in order to optimize the use of the new equipment and increase public credibility;

- The creation of examination centres equipped with sophisticated DI devices (radiotherapy, nuclear medicine, tomography, DA, NMR, etc.) and accessible to all public and private radiologists;

- Priority development of echographic techniques which have special importance for developing countries (e.g. systematic detection of such diseases as hydatidosis); and

- The general development of diagnostic procedures in order to make them more precise, short and less costly.

TURKEY

Information provided by the competent authorities of Turkey on the number of medical imaging devices in use is presented in table V.18.

Table V.18.   Medical imaging devices in use in Turkey (1980-1985)

Device type	Total in use		Number of examinations 1985
	1980	1985	
X-ray devices	594	634	2 397 789
Gamma camera	2	7	...
Ultrasound	5	16	23 593

Source: Permanent Mission of Turkey to the United Nations Office at Geneva.

UNION OF SOVIET SOCIALIST REPUBLICS

In answer to the ECE questionnaire, the competent USSR authorities provided the information given below.

Safety legislation and standards

The basic document, regulating the acceptable level of ionizing radiation emitted by medical equipment and systems and absorbed by the patient, is NRB-76 "Standards on radiation safety". All diagnostic methods and devices based on the utilization of radioactive substances and other sources of ionizing radiation must receive the prior approval of the USSR Ministry of Health. The installation and use of such devices is regulated by the "Basic sanitary regulations on work with radioactive substances and other sources of ionizing radiation". These two documents are used particularly in the field of nuclear medicine and roentgenology.

The checking of digital imaging systems used in nuclear medicine and roentgenology is strictly regulated by State standards (GOST) and sectoral standards (OST), as follows:

- X-ray and radiometric devices - methods and means of testing;

- Dosimetric and radiometric instruments - testing methods; and

- Subdivision of radiodiagnostic devices - safety requirements.

For the definition of technical characteristics and testing of DI devices and systems, the following standards are used:

- X-ray medical apparatus - general technical conditions;

- Medical diagnosis ultrasound devices (echo-pulsing, scanning) - general technical requirements and testing methods; and

- Medical diagnosis ultrasound devices - nomenclature of quality indicators.

Research and development

R and D tasks in the field of digital imaging for medical purposes receiving Government support, include:

- Digital X-ray systems for use in operating rooms and in pediatry and mammography;

- DA systems with microprocessor control;

- CT scanners for brain and body investigation;

- Multidetecting gamma CT for dynamic brain investigation;

- Mobile gamma camera with microprocessor control;

- SPET systems for body investigation;

- PET systems;

- MRI devices;

- Ultrasound devices for diagnosis of multi-gland diseases;

- Digital echo-tomoscopes with microprocessor control;

- Automated systems for processing and recording radioisotope images;

- System for analysis of X-ray images; and

- Scientific, technological, organizational and methodological principles of designing problem-oriented data bases in nuclear medicine.

International co-operation

The USSR participates actively in the scientific and technological co-operation programmes of the countries members of the Council for Mutual Economic Assistance (CMEA) established in the fields mentioned above.

UNITED KINGDOM

Information concerning the state of the art in the field of digital imaging in health care in the United Kingdom was prepared by the Department of Health and Social Security (DHSS). Some data, as well as comments on the text of the present study, were provided by the School of Medicine, University College, London.

Table V.19 shows the number of medical imaging devices in use in the United Kingdom.

Table V.19. **Medical imaging devices in use in the United Kingdom (1980-1990)**

Device type	Number of units in use			Number of examinations 1985
	1980	1985	1990*	
Film-based X-ray	2 350	2 400	2 450	23.4 million
Fluoroscopic X-ray	1 380	1 400	1 425	1.4 million
DA	-	33	70	2 375
CT scanner	61	126	200	350 000
Gamma camera	180	320	450	)
SPET	20	50	75	) 420 000
PET	1	2	4	)
MRI	1	11	40	6 000
Ultrasound	385	1 155	2 200	1.1 million
PACS	-	-	5	-

Source: N. Slark, Diagnostic Imaging, Scientific and Technical Branch of the DHSS.

Safety legislation and standards

There are no specific safety standards for DI. National and international safety standards exist for a wide range of medical equipment and IEC 601/1 (BSI 5724 Part 1) would be applied to DI equipment in medicine where appropriate. Where equipment is designed to other standards, provision is made in DHSS Document TRS 86 to cover any special requirements in the medical field.

Purchasing policy and DI assessment

In the United Kingdom, decisions regarding the choice of equipment or the need for DI are made at Regional Health Authority level. Central Government in the form of the Scientific and Technical Branch of DHSS provides advice and recommendations but does not dictate a policy on DI provisioning.

Digital imaging equipment may be purchased by direct purchase through the Regional or District Supplies Departments.

The DHSS publishes a series of reports (known as the "Blue Cover" series) which cover the assessment of a wide range of medical imaging equipment, some of which could be classified as DI equipment.

Companies active in the field

As shown in table V.20, five companies are at present involved in the production and supply of DI equipment.

Table V.20. Companies active in the DI field
in the United Kingdom

Company	Main activity
Nodecrest	Nuclear medicine (NM)
Link Systems	NM
IGEMS	NM, CT, MRI
Quantel	X-ray equipment
Picker	MRI

Source: DHSS, London 1986.

Nodecrest is a small private company totally committed to DI, mainly in the nuclear medicine and radiotheraphy treatment planning fields.

Link Systems and Quantel are individual companies within the UEI Group.

While Link Systems' main interests lie in the micro-analysis area, about 20 per cent of their effort is in DI in the field of nuclear medicine.

Quantel's main involvement is in the area of commercial DI, TV-displays, etc. They do, however, have a small interest in the medical field in the area of digital X-ray imaging.

IGEMS - International General Electric Medical Systems is a large United States based transnational company which has a small manufacturing site in the United Kingdom. This site is used for the development and production of DI equipment mainly for nuclear medicine, although some of the technology is used in the CT and MRI equipment manufactured in the United States.

Picker International Ltd., was a large company in the United States that was purchased by the United Kingdom GEC company some years ago.

At the United Kingdom site, it carries out some of the development and production of their MRI equipment. The United Kingdom company has a number of R and D partnerships with hospitals and the DHSS, mainly in the field of MRI at Hammersmith Hospital and at Nottingham.

Research and development

The DHSS continues to support the development of MRI, and the United Kingdom Department of Trade and Industry also supports a number of companies in the development of DI in medicine in the fields of NM, CT, MRI etc.

As regards available public funding, no specific amount is directly available for the development of DI.

UNITED STATES

The competent authorities of the United States, in particular the Department of Commerce, have provided continuous support to the present study. In view of United States advanced research and development in the DI field, manufacturing and implementation experience, as well as the available know-how, most of the contributions have already been incorporated in other chapters. Selected statistical data on the production and international trade in irradiation and electromedical equipment are presented below (see tables V.21, V.22 and V.23).

Table V.21. Value of shipments of irradiation and electromedical equipment in the United States (1980-1985)

Product group	Value of shipments (millions of US dollars)					
	1980	1981	1982	1983	1984	1985
X-ray and other irradiation equipment	800.0	1 003.8	1 342.2	1 543.5	1 757.7	1 631.3
Electromedical equipment	1 612.7	1 936.9	2 419.1	2 556.8	2 675.2	2 704.1
Total	2 412.7	2 940.7	3 761.3	4 100.3	4 432.9	4 335.4

Source: Current industrial reports: "Electromedical Equipment and Irradiation Equipment (including X-ray), 1985; MA 36R(85)-1 United States Department of Commerce, Bureau of the Census, Washington, July 1986.

The total figures for MRI equipment presented in table V.22 could be complemented by the review of MRI installations in 1984 and 1985 (see table V.24). According to this table the number of MRI installations increased in one year by some 270 per cent (from 83 to 217 MRI devices).

Table V.22. <u>Quantity and value of shipments of selected</u>
<u>electromedical and irradiation equipment</u>
<u>in the United States (1984-1985)</u>

Product description	1984		1985		Number of companies
	Number of units	Value (thousand US dollars)	Number of units	Value (thousand US dollars)	
Irradiation equipment, including X-ray, Beta-ray, Gamma-ray, and nuclear (medical, dental, industrial and scientific)	...	1 757 692	...	1 631 301	66
of which:					
Digital radiography equipment	416	59 925	393	56 851	4
Computerized axial tomography (CT, CAT scanners)	564	666 393	506	513 235	5
Other diagnostic X-ray equipment	3 291	420 251	3 215	435 162	11
Industrial and scientific X-ray equipment, excluding Beta- and Gamma-ray equipment	2 532	52 546	2 997	61 609	11
X-ray equipment accessories	...	137 947	...	114 397	33
X-ray tubes (sold separately)	57 282	158 582	61 252	171 877	14
Parts for X-ray equipment (sold separately)	...	26 432	...	28 267	12
All other irradiation equipment, including Beta- and Gamma-ray equipment	...	235 616	...	249 903	...
Electromedical diagnostic, therapeutic, and patient monitoring equipment, except irradiation equipment	...	2 675 193	...	2 704 077	133
of which:					
Ultrasonic scanning devices	9 046	294 220	5 172	186 755	11
MRI	145	81 226	287	154 752	5
All other diagnostic equipment (ECG, EEG, EMG, etc.)	...	430 136	...	411 384	...
Electromedical therapeutic equipment (pacemakers, electrosurgical, dialyzers, etc.)	...	919 240	...	845 637	...
Patient monitoring equipment (intensive/coronary care, perinatal, respiratory, etc.)	...	576 794	...	641 116	...
Other electromedical equipment (surgical support systems, parts and accessories sold separately)	...	373 577	...	464 433	...

Source: As for table V.21.

- 130 -

Table V.23. Shipments, exports, imports and apparent consumption
of irradiation and electromedical equipment in the
United States (1984 and 1985)

| Product group | Year | Thousand US dollars | | | Exports/Shipments (percentage) | Thousand US dollars | | Imports/apparent consumption (percentage) |
| | | Manufacturers shipments | Exports | | | Imports | Apparent consumption | |
			Value at port	Producers value				
X-ray and other irradiation equipment	1984	1 757 692	275 878	226 882	13	486 380	2 017 190	24
	1985	1 631 301	269 425	221 575	14	547 238	1 956 964	28
Electromedical equipment	1984	2 675 193	823 241	677 033	25	400 705	2 398 865	17
	1985	2 704 077	891 890	733 490	27	573 197	2 543 784	23
Total	1984	4 432 885	1 099 119	903 915	20	887 085	4 416 055	20
	1985	4 335 378	1 161 315	955 065	22	1 120 435	4 500 748	25

Source: Same as for table V.21.

Table V.24. Number of magnetic resonance imaging units
installed in the United States (1984-1985)

| Company (producer/supplier) | Number of MRI units installed | |
	1984 a/	1985 a/
Technicare	31	64
Diasonics	18	35
Siemens	7	33
GE	3	30
Picker	11	29
Fonar	5	14
Philips	4	6
Bruker	2	4
Elscint	2	2
Total units installed	83	217

Source: Diagnostic Imaging, 1986.

a/ As on 1 October of the respective year.

Companies active in the field

ADAC Laboratories focus on three product lines: (1) gamma cameras, nuclear medicine DIP systems, PET (2) digital fluorography, nuclear emission CT scanners (3) radiation therapy planning, RIS. In the field of DA, manufacturing agreements were signed with Picker International (as from 1981) and Fischer Imaging (1982 only). 1985 revenues reached some $US 57 million.

Advanced Technical Laboratories (ATL) manufacture diagnostic ultrasonic equipment, combining a wide variety of features for cardiac, obstetrical, abdominal, vascular, radiological and intra-operative applications. 1984 sales were estimated at $US 105 million.

Diasonics sales in 1985 were $US 158 million. The company is a market leader in DI/ultrasound equipment (including cardiological ultrasound). The second area of concentration is X-ray equipment (in 1983 Fischer Imaging Corporation was acquired). Finally, Diasonics manufacture MRI scanning equipment (first company to use superconductive magnets). Manufacturing facilities are located in the United States, Europe, Japan and Australia.

Fonar specializes in the manufacture of whole-body medical scanning equipment. In 1984, an R and D agreement was signed with Soft Sheen Products to develop MRI scanners employing non-superconductive magnets.

General Electric Company, one of the world's largest and most diversified industrial corporations, was incorporated in 1892. Its Medical Systems Division, which is active in all the imaging modalities, is currently increasing its interests, including the establishment of its own plant to build superconductive magnets. Non-DI products include all types of patient-monitoring equipment and radiology supplies. Division sales in 1984 were cited at $US 715 million.

Hewlett-Packard, a major designer and manufacturer of measurement and computer technology, is also active in medical electronics. Main product lines lie outside DI equipment. However, its Medical Products Group also manufactures ultrasonic imaging equipment.

Johnson & Johnson Ultrasound is a subsidiary of Johnson & Johnson Inc., one of the world's largest manufacturers of health-care (and other) products. Johnson & Johnson Ultrasound specializes in ultrasound imagers, cardiac imaging instruments, medical transducers and ultrasonic couplants. It also distributes the ultrasound products of the Japanese Aloka Company.

Technicare is a wholly-owned subsidiary of Johnson & Johnson (acquired from Ohio Nuclear in 1979). Its revenues were estimated at $US 270 million in 1983. Technicare manufactures a wide range of DI equipment, including CT head and body scanners, nuclear medicine cameras, DA systems, ultrasonic scanners and MRI devices (these were among the first approved by the FDA in 1984). Technicare undertakes international co-operation in eight European countries, as well as in Australia and Hong Kong.

Research and development

Little statistical information is available on R and D in the area of
medical equipment and even less in that of DI equipment. It is estimated that
the Federal Government and companies producing medical devices provide
financial support to R and D amounting to some 3 per cent of the value of
manufacturers shipments (R and D expenditure of industry as a whole amounted
to 2.4 per cent of shipments in 1980). Companies active in the field of
medical diagnostic imaging indicate that R and D expenditures in this area can
attain a figure three times as high as the 3 per cent mentioned above.

The National Institute of Health (NIH) supports intramural and extramural
R and D in MRI technology. The National Cancer Institute (NCI) has been
supporting R and D in biomedical applications of MRI, including
MRI spectroscopy and the use of MRI in the study of metabolism of both normal
and cancer cells. In the past, NIH has supported MRI spectroscopic research
at various locations in the United States.

The 1984 OTA Report on Nuclear Magnetic Resonance Imaging Technology
states that NIH is currently making availabe some $US 2 million for
MRI related research at various institutions.

While the National Science Foundation (NSF) has in the past supported
pioneering research of MRI imaging at the University of California at
Berkeley, it has no programmes in that area at present. The Federal
Government supports over 52 per cent of total health R and D. Approximately
70 per cent of this comes from grants and funding from NIH. Under current
budgetary considerations, the Government is planning to rescind funding for
nearly 600 NIH grants in 1986.

The Federal Government of the United States is currently launching an
evaluation programme on digital imaging in health care. It has selected
three test sites (University of Washington, Georgetown University and
George Washington University). The next step is to select vendors to supply
the equipment and systems. Installations will take place late in 1987.
Evaluations will take three years.

CHAPTER VI - LIKELY TRENDS IN THE APPLICATION OF DIGITAL IMAGING

1. NEW TECHNICAL DEVELOPMENTS

1.1 The digital imaging field in general

The personal-computer market is preparing the ground for computer-assisted medical diagnosis systems. Physicians are increasingly using them for more complex tasks, and becoming familiar with this technology. It can be expected that the efficient use of computer technology (both hardware and software) will result in several significant changes, providing faster diagnosis with greater specificity while using less-invasive or non-invasive techniques, with more information being available through improved communication systems.

For the advancement of DI technologies, certain breakthroughs are needed. Table VI.1 summarizes the identified problem areas for DI devices. It is based on the material presented in chapter II in the discussion of the state of the art.

Although the emphasis in table VI.1 is seemingly on technical problems, clinical and socio-economic studies that investigate the clinical capabilities and restrictions of imaging technologies and their impact on the delivery of health care are equally important.

1.2 Man/machine interfaces [76]

The successful introduction of PACS in hospitals will decisively depend on the user interfaces, i.e. image stations. Severe user acceptance problems must be solved if the clinical work procedures of medical-image interpretation and consultation are to be based on electronic display systems instead of using the traditional photographic films and lightboxes. Image work-stations will be the principal and critical interaction devices for radiologists to access, process and communicate information. PACS will be technically very complex. The design of image work-stations has to focus on solutions for man/machine interfaces that protect the users from involvement in the technical details and that fit into the organization of the radiology departments and adapt to the various clinical tasks and to the users.

Figure VI.1 illustrates the interaction of the DI process with the attitudes and motivation of the radiologist. If the DWS does not adapt to this process, the willingness and involvement of the clinicians could be in danger.

User-friendly communication is mandatory. Some changes to the work practices of the users seem unavoidable. However, it must be remembered that image work-stations will only be accepted if their use is as convenient, fast and accurate as with the conventional film/lightbox system and if they offer some improvements or additional features.

Table VI.1. Areas identified for R and D in digital imaging technologies

DI device	Specific R and D area
X-ray	
Digital radiography	Transducing and geometry
CT scanner	Speed
Digital subtraction angiography	Resolution
Nuclear medicine	
Gamma camera	Stable technology
SPECT	Transducing and geometry
Positron Emission Tomography	Tracer kinetic models
	Radiopharmaceuticals (positron emitters)
	Compact cyclotron
	Clinical applications
MRI	
Magnetic resonance imaging	See table II.12
US	
Ultrasound	Transmission ultrasound
	Tissue characterization
	Combined B-mode/Doppler in real-time
PACS	
Diagnostic workstation	Man/machine interface
	Speed
	Three-dimensional/projections and visualization
	Image handling and interpretation
Local Area Networks	Speed (throughput)
	Protocols/standards
Archive	Laser disk technology
New areas	
Radiotherapy	Computer-aided radiotherapy (see figure II.13)
Microwave imaging	Basic research (possibly breast cancer screening)
Microscope analysis	Image interpretation

Figure VI.1.   Process of diagnostic imaging
               (work routines and clinician attitudes)

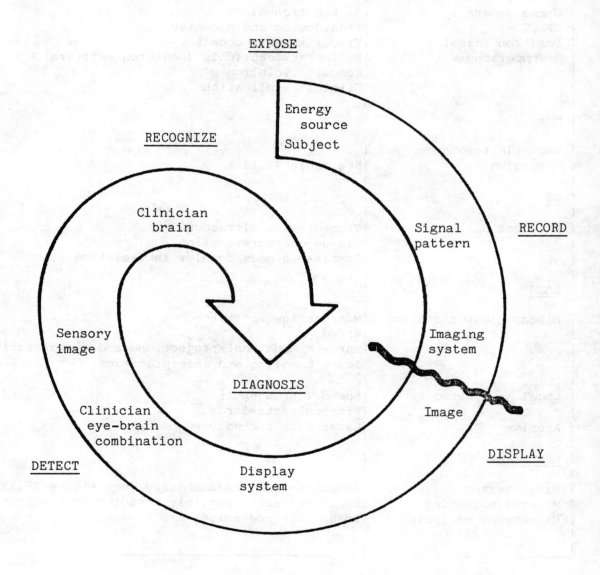

Source: CAR '85 - International Symposium and Exhibition on Computer
         Assisted Radiology, Berlin, June 1985. Proceedings.

1.3 Image processing and interpretation

Image processing and interpretation algorithms applicable to the specific medical imaging modalities are in a relatively early stage of development. There are many simple filtering algorithms that can be used to "cosmetically polish" the images (removal of distortion, edge enhancement, contour detection etc.). Before image processing and the interpretation algorithms can be effectively utilized, several different approaches must be developed, verified and evaluated, in close collaboration with the users.

Image interpretation is based on recognized patterns (features). It is the decision-making process the physician goes through when reviewing the images and the additional information about the patient that is available to him and arriving at a diagnostic conclusion. Expert systems technology (a sub-field of artificial intelligence) offers a way to automate this process. R and D in expert systems is at present extremely active and should in a few years result in efficient expert systems development environments that will make this technology commercially successful.

In order to apply the expert systems technology to the interpretation of medical images, the knowledge and decision process of physicians interpreting images must be formalized into the expert system.

1.4 Network developments

For communication of medical images one needs (1) an agreement on the format of representation of the digital image data; (2) a communication protocol; and (3) a high-speed local area network (LAN) within the hospital and some other means of communicating images at greater distances.

As already discussed briefly in chapter II.7, the American College of Radiology (ACR) and the National Electrical Manufacturers Association (NEMA) have prepared an "ACR-NEMA Digital Imaging and Communications Standard" based on the Open Systems Interconnect (OSI) protocol. The standard is intended to be used as illustrated in figure VI.2. It specifies the image representation format and the communication protocol.

The ACR-NEMA image format contains the following information:

- Identification data of the patient;

- Data of the examination and imaging device used;

- Other relational data (related images etc.);

- Image representation data (co-ordinates of the imaging device and patient in relation to the images so that further processing and comparison of images is possible); and

- Image pixel data.

The transmission protocol was presented briefly in chapter II.8 (figure II.24). It is based on the OSI transport layer standard. Since manufacturers of DI devices do not have in-house capabilities for computers or microcomputers, the communication protocols they adopt will be based on those

Figure VI.2.   Location of the ACR-NEMA standard interface

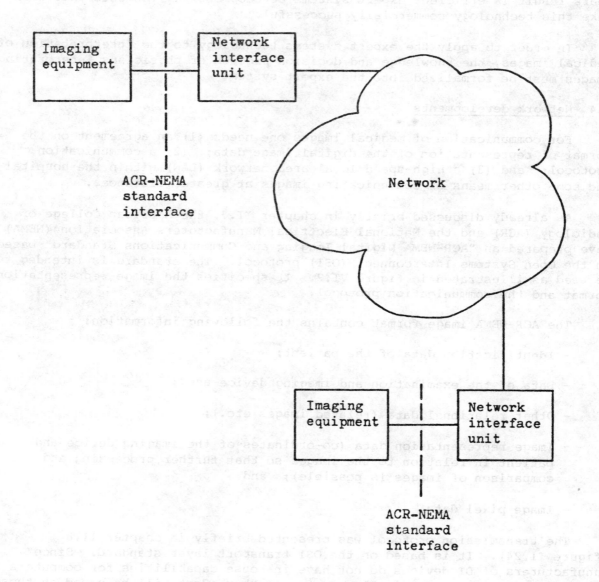

Source: ACR-NEMA Digital Imaging and Communications Standard,
         1 July 1985.   Available from the Manager, Engineering Dept.,
         NEMA, 2101 L Street, N.W., Washington D.C. 20037.

available and supported by the computer manufacturers. At the moment there are several standards available, of which the ones based on IEEE 802.3 and 802.4 are the most used. However, given the nature of recent developments, it is difficult to forecast what the final standards are going to be.

The transmission speeds obtainable with present LANs are not high enough for an imaging department to be interconnected with PACS. At most, images can be transferred between disks at 1 Mbit/s in a local area network. Transmission of a normal CT image (512 x 512 pixel, 12 bit) would take three seconds. Fibre optics are still very expensive, although capable of the required speed. A much higher speed is in particular required between the intermediate storage and the DWS (see figure VI.3).

2. ESTIMATES OF THE GROWTH OF DIGITAL IMAGING INSTALLATIONS

Growth projections for medical imaging devices are discussed in chapter II.9. Similar projections for PACS are not available. It can be expected that the utilization of the available imaging modalities will in future be quite different from the present situation, taking into account that, within the next few years, certain changes will take place, namely:

- There is room for considerable technical improvements in some of the imaging modalities (especially MRI and PET), and the basic technologies necessary for PACS will mature;

- The clinical applications and indications for use of each imaging modality will be subject to continuous evolution and evaluation;

- The cost-effectiveness of various imaging modalities and their impact on health-care delivery will be the subject of continuing investigation.

To make estimates at this stage on the desired optimum or saturation levels for DI devices is impossible.

As indicated in chapter II.9 (see also annexes III, IV and V) the whole field of electromedical equipment seems very promising as concerns the growth of international trade. Namely, the increased use of various types of new and innovated diagnostic devices and systems, quite often interrelated with the introduction of medical information systems (MIS, HIS, RIS), can contribute significantly to effective health-care services in the ECE region. In this respect, the experience acquired from the increasing number of successful pilot installations (diagnostic units and centres, computerization of hospitals, etc.) may well serve in advocating sophisticated (however still costly) solutions for current health-care problems.

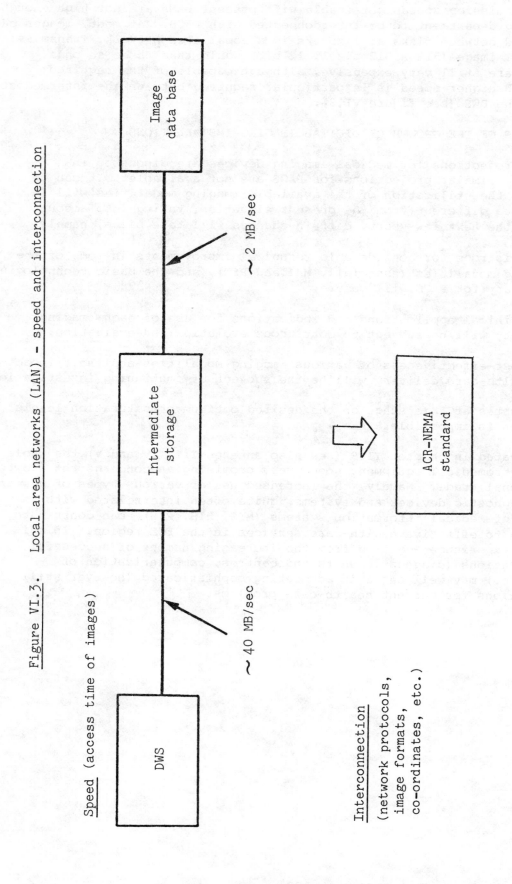

Figure VI.3. Local area networks (LAN) – speed and interconnection

Speed (access time of images)

DWS

~ 40 MB/sec

Intermediate storage

~ 2 MB/sec

Image data base

Interconnection
(network protocols,
image formats,
co-ordinates, etc.)

ACR-NEMA standard

Source: Medical Engineering Laboratory,
Technical Research Centre of Finland.

CHAPTER VII - INTERNATIONAL CO-OPERATION IN THE FIELD OF DIGITAL IMAGING

1. INTERNATIONAL STANDARDS

Terminology for the DI field in general and for its medical applications in particular has not been established. The International Electrotechnical Commission (IEC) has published a vocabulary on radiology, [77] but it does not cover the latest developments. Consequently, the terms used vary, e.g. CT and CAT (computed axial tomography) and MRI and NMR. In the drafting of international standards for the DI field, terminology must also be standardized.

For the image format several possibilities exist, of which the ACR-NEMA standard seems to be the most promising, since it is complete, covering also the transmission protocol section, and since it is based on the OSI transport layer standard developed by ISO. For image formats and interfaces, those manufacturers that have a more complete line of DI products can offer their own solutions. For the future advancement of DI in medicine, it should be in everybody's interest to ensure the development of an international image format and transmission standard that is also supported by the computer manufacturers.

Man/machine interfaces are an area where much effort is needed. It is not proposed that these should be standardized in the near future. On the contrary, man/machine interfaces will probably be one of the key competitive factors in the future. Co-operation in this field should use the experiences of such fields as ergonomy, visualization techniques, design of control panels and keyboards etc.

The users of medical DI devices would benefit greatly if disclosure standards were available for the imaging devices. IEC's Technical Committee TC62 on electromedical equipment is working towards that end. For the time being it has, however, set a higher priority on the preparation of safety standards for electromedical equipment.

2. QUALITY AND PERFORMANCE ASSURANCE, TESTING AND SAFETY

In the design and production of DI devices, besides their internal production standards, companies use those international and national requirements that are applicable to the product in question. Normally these consist of safety requirements and of Good Manufacturing Practices (GMP). In some countries, certain products must be tested and approved before they can be marketed (premarket approval). Although international government trade agreements try to remove barriers to trade, the national requirements for medical equipment are as yet far from being harmonized.

Quality-assurance (QA) procedures aim at keeping the device in optimum working condition. For certain medical imaging devices, national organizations have developed QA procedures. These are normally based on periodic checks of the image quality using image phantoms and on preventive maintenance. Such procedures exist for film-based X-ray [78] and gamma cameras. [79] Image phantoms also exist for other modalities.

A wider use of these QA procedures and phantoms is advocated on the international level by respective scientific societies and WHO, since not only do they improve image quality but they also reduce the use of materials and, most important, provide the users with means to control equipment functioning, resulting in improved staff motivation.

3.   PATENTS AND LICENSING

A number of patents in DI are held by individuals, companies and investment groups. For the present study, no special attempts have been made to collect information on the number and types of patents and licence agreements relevant to this field.

One concern regarding patents is that they might create undesirable barriers to entry into the DI field. Data available on the MRI field, however, suggests that patents have not created such a barrier. [80] Other problems could be the stifling of prompt dissemination of scientific discoveries in order to provide time for filing patents, and the redirection of the focus of university-based research from basic science to the development of patentable devices and techniques. The existence of a large number of collaborative research relationships between industry, universities and research institutions suggest that these concerns are not valid either.

4.   WAYS AND MEANS OF STRENGTHENING INTERNATIONAL CO-OPERATION

Co-operation could be strengthened through industrial, government and scientific interests. Company interests in co-operation are limited, since they have to protect their own technologies in order to maintain or increase their market positions. Safety, image format and communication protocol standards are the areas of exception. On the other hand, R and D investments needed to enter the DI field are considerable. Companies may therefore see advantages in co-operating on a pre-competition level for the development of technologies that they can use in product development. An example of this is the Nordic R and D programme on Computer-Aided Radiotherapy (CART) (see figure II.13). [81]

Government interests can deal with improving either the circumstances in which the companies operate or the cost-effectiveness of health care. Studies from the technological viewpoint, similar to the present one, should be carried out regularly by integovernmental agencies and United Nations regional economic commissions such as ECE and other international organizations on areas in medical equipment technology where rapid development is taking place and where it will have an impact on both the industry and health care. To obtain information on the clinical applications, indications for use and cost-effectiveness of new technologies, co-operation is also necessary. The Regional Office for Europe of WHO has been active in this area and has organized and supported several meetings. The newly-established International Society of Technology Assessment in Health Care with its journal will be a good channel for gathering and disseminating information.

Co-operation on the scientific level is traditionally strong. At the moment there are many international organizations that are active in DI. Some of these are listed in table VII.1.

The BAZIS (Central Development and Support Group Hospital Information System) of the Leiden University Hospital, which is also the site of the secretariat of EuroPACS, is collecting information on ongoing PACS research and development activities in Europe, the United States and Japan. [82]

The European situation is presented in the Newsletters of EuroPACS. [83] The latest situation in the United States was reported in a paper presented to the Fifth World Congress on Medical Informatics - MEDINFO '86 - in Washington D.C. in October 1986. [84] A report on the state of the art in Japan will be available following a study tour which is scheduled for May 1987.

Most of the organizations listed in table VII.1 have their own journals publishing scientific articles, and organize conferences, symposia and meetings (see annex VIII). The efficient use by government organizations of the resources and channels provided by these organizations should be encouraged.

Table VII.1. International organizations that have an interest in digital imaging

	Battelle Memorial Institute
ECE	United Nations Economic Commission for Europe - Working Party on Engineering Industries and Automation
EFMI	European Federation for Medical Informatics
EFOMP	European Federation of Organizations in Medical Physics
	European Society of Magnetic Resonance in Medicine and Biology
ESR	European Society on Radiology
EuroPACS	European PACS Society
FDI	International Dental Federation
IAMLT	International Association of Medical Laboratory Technologists
IBI	The Institute of Biomedical Information
	International Bio-Medical Information Service
ICRP	International Commission on Radiological Protection
ICRU	International Commission on Radiation Units and Measurements
IEC	International Electrotechnical Commission
IFAC	International Federation of Automatic Control
IFIP	International Federation for Information Processing
IFMBE	International Federation for Medical and Biological Engineering
IFORS	International Federation for Operational Research Societies
IIASA	International Institute of Applied Systems Analysis
IIMEBE	International Institute for Medical Electronics and Biological Engineering
IMEKO	International Measurement Confederation
IMIA	International Medical Informatics Association
INICR	International Non-Ionizing Radiation Commission
IOMP	International Organization for Medical Physics
IRPA	International Radiation Protection Association
ISCEV	International Society for Clinical Electrophysiology of Vision
ISFC	International Society and Federation of Cardiology
ISMR	International Society for Magnetic Resonance
ISNM	International Society for Nuclear Medicine
ISO	International Organization for Standardization
ISR	International Society on Radiology
ISTAHC	International Society of Technology Assessment in Health Care
IUPESM	International Union of Physical and Engineering Sciences in Medicine
WHO	World Health Organization
WFUMB	World Federation of Ultrasound in Medicine and Biology

CONCLUSIONS

The conclusions that can be drawn from the present study are the
following:

(1) Digital imaging (DI) is a highly interdisciplinary field applying
numerous basic technologies that are being developed mainly independently
of the medical DI interests.

(2) DI comprises image sources of which the most important are for diagnostic
imaging (digital radiology, digital angiography, CT scanning, diagnostic
ultrasound, nuclear imaging, positron-emission tomography and magnetic
resonance imaging) and a picture archiving and communication system
(PACS) for image-processing purposes.

(3) The field of DI is at present advancing very rapidly owing to recent
innovations in imaging possibilities and the fast developments taking
place in information technology (mainly computers, computer software,
local area networks and network protocols).

(4) Within a few years it will be technically possible and economically
feasible to build clinical imaging departments that are totally digital,
i.e. do not rely on film as a storage medium.

(5) The new imaging modalities are non-invasive or less traumatic than the
old ones. They seem to be safer, since they do not use ionizing
radiation to obtain information. Also, they hold the promise of more
accurate and faster diagnosing capabilities than the old methods. Their
capacity in handling patients is larger, owing to the extensive use of
computer technology and because the clinical procedures for obtaining
images are less time consuming. On the other hand, since they are
complex, they are more expensive to buy and maintain than the old imaging
devices. The operating costs of these devices cannot as yet be
accurately calculated or estimated because neither the device technology
nor the clinical applications and indications for use have so far
stabilized.

(6) For the industry, this situation is potentially very lucrative. The
market potential is large. It is expected that the purchase price will
not be the most important factor in competing for the markets. More
emphasis will instead be on image quality and product capabilities
together with effectiveness, reliability and life-cycle costs. This will
require more investments in R and D and closer co-operation with
university- and hospital-based research.

(7) Health-care providers are at present trying to introduce cost-containment
measures in order to achieve a better control of health-care costs. This
will result in more careful analysis, evaluation and assessment of new
medical technologies before they can be adopted, to make sure that they
improve the overall cost-effectiveness of health care.

(8) In the case of DI, this means that the rate of diffusion of new
technologies will depend on these assessment and evaluation studies.

(9) Health-care personnel using DI devices will require additional training.
     There will also be some fundamental changes in the types of jobs
     available in DI.

(10) The present study cannot predict the diffusion of DI technology in health
     care. At one extreme, it could be distributed to the primary level and,
     at the other, centralized to larger hospitals. Another open question is
     whether the imaging modalities will be managed by one single medical
     speciality (radiology) or be fragmented and shared between several
     medical specialities.

(11) The drive towards cost-containment will cause problems for the industry,
     resulting in acquisitions and mergers. The rapidly expanding role of
     data and image processing will be a major challenge to the X-ray
     equipment manufacturers at present dominating the field. The extent to
     which they are able to respond will decide how concentrated or fragmented
     the market will be in the future.

(12) Considerable difficulties have been encountered in making this study,
     owing to the dynamic development of the field. Detailed up-to-date
     statistics on DI equipment and systems are not available. Those that
     have been used are two to three years old and, furthermore, their
     reliability is in some cases questionable. Assessment reports on
     clinical usefulness and application together with economic considerations
     are scarce and, in the case of some modalities, non-existent.

(13) The development of totally integrated digital imaging departments should
     go hand in hand with the practical evaluation of such departments. For
     digital imaging departments, the other clinical data will also have to be
     computerized. These investments will be sizeable. Collaborative,
     cost-sharing efforts are therefore needed to keep expenditure down to a
     reasonable level.

Annexes

Annex I

SEMINARS SPONSORED BY THE ECE WORKING PARTY ON ENGINEERING
INDUSTRIES AND AUTOMATION (1971-1987) AND ITS PREDECESSORS

Title, place and date of seminar	Symbol of report
1. Application of Computers as an Aid to Management, Geneva (Switzerland), 11-15 October 1971	AUTOMATION/Working Paper No.3
2. Application of Metal and Non-Metal Materials in Engineering Industries, Varna (Bulgaria), 28 May-1 June 1973	ENGIN/SEM.1/2
3. Application of Numerically Controlled Machine Tools, Prague (Czechoslovakia), 12-17 November 1973	AUTOMAT/SEM.1/3
4. Automated Industrial Production, its Social and Economic Consequences, Lyon (France), 16-21 September 1974	AUTOMAT/SEM.2/2
5. Techno-Economic Aspects and Results of Anti-Corrosion Measures in Engineering Industries, Geneva (Switzerland), 27-31 January 1975	ENGIN/SEM.2/2
6. Use of Automated Process Control Systems in Industry, Moscow (USSR), 26-31 May 1975	AUTOMAT/SEM.3/2
7. Automated Integrated Production Systems in Mechanical Engineering, Prague (Czechoslovakia), 1-6 November 1976	AUTOMAT/SEM.4/2
8. Industrial Robots and Programmable Logical Controllers, Copenhagen (Denmark), 5-7 September 1977	AUTOMAT/SEM.5/2
9. Engineering Equipment for Foundries and Advanced Methods for Production of such Equipment, Geneva (Switzerland), 28 November-3 December 1977	ENGIN/SEM.3/2
10. Techno-Economic Trends in Airborne Equipment for Agriculture and Other Selected Areas of the National Economy (AERO-AGRO '78), Warsaw (Poland), 18-22 September 1978	ENGIN/SEM.4/3
11. Computer-Aided Design Systems as an Integrated Part of Industrial Production, Geneva (Switzerland), 14-18 May 1979	AUTOMAT/SEM.6/2
12. Development and Use of Industrial Handling Equipment, Sofia (Bulgaria), 3-8 September 1979	ENGIN/SEM.5/2

Title, place and date of seminar	Symbol of report
13. Innovation in Engineering Industries: Techno-Economic Aspects of Fabrication Processes and Quality Control, Turin (Italy), 9-13 June 1980	ENGIN/SEM.6/3
14. Automation of Welding, Kiev (Ukrainian SSR), 13-17 October 1980	AUTOMAT/SEM.7/3
15. Automation of Assembly in Engineering Industries, Geneva (Switzerland), 22-25 September 1981	AUTOMAT/SEM.8/3
16. Present Use and Prospects for Precision Measuring Instruments in Engineering Industries, Dresden (German Democratic Republic), 20-24 September 1982	ENG.AUT/SEM.1/3
17. Innovation in Biomedical Equipment, Budapest (Hungary), 2-6 May 1983	ENG.AUT/SEM.2/3
18. Flexible Manufacturing Systems - Design and Applications, Sofia (Bulgaria), 24-28 September 1984	ENG.AUT/SEM.3/4
19. Development and Use of Powder Metallurgy in Engineering Industries, Minsk (Byelorussian SSR), 25-29 March 1985	ENG.AUT/SEM.4/3
20. Industrial Robotics '86 - International Experience, Developments and Applications, Brno (Czechoslovakia), 24-28 February 1986	ENG.AUT/SEM.5/4
21. Automation Means in Preventive Medicine '87, Piestany (Czechoslovakia), 28 September-2 October 1987	ENG.AUT/SEM.6/...

PROVISIONAL PROGRAMME FOR THE ECE SEMINAR ON
AUTOMATION MEANS IN PREVENTIVE MEDICINE '87
(Piestany, Czechoslovakia, 28 September-2 October 1987)

SECTION I

Technical and medical aspects of preventive treatment

(a)   Interaction between developments in health care and innovations in
      medical engineering (e.g. national contributions)

(b)   Symptomatology - determination of optimum number and types of
      diagnostic indicators

(c)   Diagnostic systems for various diseases and types of preventive
      treatment

(d)   Universality of diagnostic systems, equipment and components -
      technical, operational and organizational barriers

SECTION II

Design, production and use of equipment for preventive medical treatment

(a)   Digital image processing (DIP) equipment and systems (various X-ray
      technologies, computer tomography, nuclear medicine, ultrasound,
      magnetic resonance imaging, etc.)

(b)   Other advanced instruments, equipment and systems for preventive
      diagnostics and screening programmes (bioelectric recording
      equipment, clinical monitoring equipment, cell and blood analysis,
      biosensors, apparatus for individual use, etc.)

(c)   Computerization of diagnostic information processes (software means
      and expert diagnostic systems, archiving and communication systems,
      integration aspects, etc.)

(d)   Application experience in various areas and at different levels of
      use (screening programmes, diagnostic centres, laboratory
      tests, etc.)

SECTION III

Economic and social considerations

(a)   Economic evaluation (cost/benefit implications, quality assurance
      and reliability, various support programmes, criteria of
      efficiency, etc.)

(b) Social and related aspects (improvement of health services, safety, patient involvement, etc.)

(c) Standardization and unification (modularity, compatibility and versatility, terminology, etc.)

(d) Preventive maintenance and repair of medical and related equipment, including computing, measuring and controlling devices

(e) Training and education of personnel for the selection and optimum use of appropriate medical technology

SECTION IV

International co-operation

(a) Prerequisites for international trade in medical equipment (marketing methods, competitiveness, sales strategies, etc.)

(b) Role of the international division of labour in the field of medical engineering (research and design, technology transfer and licensing, manufacturing, services, etc.)

(c) Activities of the relevant international governmental and non-governmental organizations

---

Annex III

Exports and imports of electromedical equipment of 24 selected countries, 1978-1985

(Thousands of US dollars)

Country		1978	1979	1980	1981	1982	1983	1984	1985
Australia	Export	...	2 467	3 174	2 346	1 356	3 667	2 566	5 425
	Import	...	41 575	33 844	40 076	48 397	60 157	64 401	81 365
	Balance	...	-39 108	-30 670	-37 730	-47 041	-56 490	-61 835	-75 940
Austria	E	15 807	21 861	23 824	19 934	17 247	19 844	24 092	32 729
	I	27 958	32 763	37 589	31 689	33 928	33 942	32 279	39 287
	B	-12 151	-10 902	-13 765	-11 755	-16 681	-14 098	-8 187	-6 558
Belgium and Luxembourg	E	77 095	91 009	96 806	69 603	24 560	20 185	17 906	43 294
	I	88 596	99 928	81 696	68 832	56 159	53 504	51 161	57 583
	B	-11 501	-8 919	+15 110	+ 771	-31 599	-33 319	-33 255	-14 289
Canada	E	25 180	29 595	28 855	35 015	39 325	38 636	34 150	23 120
	I	66 827	82 570	105 452	110 569	117 091	142 224	143 937	159 900
	B	-41 647	-52 975	-76 597	-75 554	-77 766	-103 588	-109 787	-136 780
Czechoslovakia	E	...	...	...	...	35 111	32 890	36 764	...
	I	...	...	...	...	31 851	34 780	38 542	...
	B	...	...	...	...	+3 260	-1 890	-1 778	...
Denmark	E	32 049	45 611	52 768	53 308	60 914	68 947	79 351	94 868
	I	18 526	27 272	22 767	17 341	17 386	18 219	22 833	25 079
	B	+13 523	+18 339	+30 001	+35 967	+43 528	+50 728	+56 518	+69 789
Finland	E	8 077	11 903	16 568	17 684	17 430	17 436	27 508	27 428
	I	11 566	13 421	18 568	18 041	15 069	19 125	21 592	25 363
	B	-3 489	-1 518	-2 000	-357	+2 361	-1 689	+5 916	+2 065
France	E	134 417	168 028	150 179	139 863	145 171	128 686	115 634	138 144
	I	142 755	182 792	149 215	157 807	165 754	142 443	163 699	166 045
	B	-8 338	-14 764	-964	-17 944	-20 583	-13 757	-48 065	-27 901

Country		1978	1979	1980	1981	1982	1983	1984	1985
Germany, Federal Republic of	Export	467 295	562 629	613 801	563 589	624 248	682 034	638 789	734 574
	Import	201 712	271 471	262 590	240 789	237 214	248 606	249 405	300 893
	Balance	+265 583	+291 158	+351 211	+322 800	+387 034	+433 428	+389 384	+433 681
Hong Kong	E	4	1	-	226	508	970	924	1 379
	I	3 045	5 001	6 131	13 470	26 908	25 951	28 010	31 556
	B	-3 041	-5 000	-6 131	-13 244	-26 400	-24 981	-27 086	-30 177
Ireland	E	1 843	4 453	3 125	9 270	1 901	12 640	3 711	1 901
	I	10 170	12 224	10 982	13 509	6 984	13 043	5 864	6 984
	B	-8 327	-7 771	-7 857	-4 239	-5 083	- 403	-2 153	-5 083
Israel	E	...	...	...	66 063	80 847	114 272	114 131	115 016
	I	...	...	...	18 956	25 409	36 770	37 965	37 506
	B	...	...	...	+47 107	+55 438	+77 502	+76 166	+77 510
Italy	E	54 078	63 155	74 981	70 726	59 705	64 833	60 324	69 443
	I	66 418	81 973	131 932	88 188	87 351	79 069	84 814	105 014
	B	-12 340	-18 818	-56 951	-17 462	-27 646	-14 236	-24 490	-35 571
Japan	E	108 289	137 450	197 368	250 619	274 161	381 857	495 739	659 423
	I	90 214	159 748	173 940	141 962	138 615	131 731	141 933	153 003
	B	+18 075	-22 298	+23 428	+108 657	+135 546	+250 126	+353 806	+506 420
Korea, Rep. of	E	1 065	1 465	1 075	974	1 376	1 374	1 911	2 145
	I	20 648	23 122	28 011	30 269	52 828	60 092	55 567	72 023
	B	-19 583	-21 657	-26 936	-29 295	-51 452	-58 718	-53 656	-69 878
Netherlands	E	232 603	285 526	288 580	288 765	295 260	275 162	296 430	347 820
	I	115 333	140 676	158 965	130 178	114 663	121 829	124 999	140 190
	B	+117 270	+144 850	+129 615	+158 587	+180 597	+153 333	+171 431	+207 630

Annex III (continued)

Country		1978	1979	1980	1981	1982	1983	1984	1985
Norway	Export	2 830	3 396	4 804	4 013	4 607	6 421	8 015	10 300
	Import	16 777	19 063	19 998	21 133	19 763	23 378	27 193	27 985
	Balance	-13 947	-15 667	-15 194	-17 120	-15 156	-16 957	-19 178	-17 685
Poland	E	...	...	...	...	12 150	13 356	12 854	...
	I	...	...	...	...	17 485	19 253	23 766	...
	B	...	...	...	...	-5 335	-5 897	-10 912	...
Singapore	E	...	1 977	2 666	3 883	4 767	3 777	5 235	7 169
	I	...	8 137	6 501	9 722	11 848	9 407	15 233	18 587
	B	...	-6 160	-3 835	-5 839	-7 081	-5 630	-9 998	-11 418
Spain	E	5 947	9 706	11 276	9 216	7 338	8 116	12 942	15 664
	I	36 851	32 390	45 035	47 338	56 289	44 814	37 392	45 677
	B	-30 904	-22 684	-33 759	-38 122	-48 951	-36 698	-24 450	-30 013
Sweden	E	73 856	96 497	114 469	102 670	95 305	92 313	84 692	109 919
	I	29 659	42 139	41 616	36 087	47 835	55 095	42 236	47 243
	B	+44 197	+54 358	+72 853	+66 583	+47 470	+37 218	+42 456	+62 676
Switzerland	E	37 210	36 997	40 055	38 686	36 299	44 624	47 675	52 171
	I	35 548	41 457	50 133	49 409	49 783	50 449	48 834	50 486
	B	+1 662	-4 460	-10 078	-10 723	-13 484	-5 825	-1 159	+1 685
United Kingdom	E	120 864	126 496	116 823	126 151	147 431	165 206	151 794	161 751
	I	81 488	103 454	115 807	139 069	159 919	156 989	142 423	136 157
	B	+39 376	+23 042	+1 016	-12 918	-12 488	+8 217	+9 371	+25 594
United States	E	511 436	698 742	813 146	983 732	1 010 276	1 068 052	1 082 632	1 149 739
	I	247 071	288 918	319 326	394 083	493 307	689 843	851 933	1 081 326
	B	+264 365	+409 824	+493 820	+589 649	+516 969	+378 209	+230 699	+68 413

Source: United Nations Statistics "Comtrade Database".

Exports and imports of electromedical equipment of selected and other reporting countries, 1978-1985

(Thousands of US dollars)

		1978	1979	1980	1981	1982	1983	1984	1985 a/
Exports of selected countries	Total value	1 909 945	2 398 965	2 668 806	2 873 779	3 023 250	3 265 297	3 355 771	3 803 422
	Number of countries	19	21	21	22	24	24	24	22
	Arithmetical mean	100 523	114 236	127 086	130 626	125 969	136 054	139 824	161 911
Exports of other reporting countries	Total value	3 091	2 968	4 793	4 119	4 304	1 085	2 351	2 448
	Number of countries	20	29	25	30	30	22	17	7
	Arithmetical mean	155	102	192	137	143	049	138	350
Imports of selected countries	Total value	1 311 162	1 710 094	1 844 729	1 844 043	2 042 797	2 270 714	2 456 011	2 809 252
	Number of countries	19	21	21	22	24	24	24	22
	Arithmetical mean	69 009	81 433	87 844	83 820	85 117	94 613	102 334	127 693
Imports of other reporting countries	Total value	125 309	143 016	246 528	310 199	340 124	164 000	102 297	23 521
	Number of countries	43	51	53	62	61	40	25	10
	Arithmetical mean	2 914	2 804	4 651	5 003	5 576	4 100	4 092	2 352

Source: United Nations Statistics "Comtrade Database".

a/ Based on a limited number of country replies.

Annex V

Exports and imports of electromedical equipment of selected countries in 1983

(Millions of US dollars)

Exporting country	Total	Bulgaria	Czechoslovakia	German Dem. Republic	Hungary	Poland	Romania	USSR	Yugoslavia	Argentina	Brazil	China	India	Mexico
Czechoslovakia	32.9	0.3	-	6.4	1.9	8.6	0.3	13.3	-	-	-	0.3	-	-
France	128.7	-	-	0.1	0.3	0.2	-	2.1	0.1	0.2	23.2	0.4	0.2	1.5
German Dem. Republic	69.0	3.5	7.5	-	7.0	5.4	3.0	38.4	0.2	-	0.2	-	-	-
Germany, Fed. Rep. of	682.0	4.8	5.3	...	3.0	4.7	1.5	18.1	8.6	1.2	3.1	10.2	5.8	3.7
Hungary	29.2	1.1	1.7	0.9	-	3.5	0.6	11.6	-	-	-	3.9	-	-
Japan	381.9	-	-	0.3	0.1	-	-	3.9	3.3	0.8	1.1	59.7	4.2	1.3
Netherlands	275.2	0.4	1.5	0.1	0.4	1.1	0.7	1.4	1.4	0.1	1.8	1.4	4.0	0.1
Poland	13.4	0.1	3.3	0.7	0.7	-	-	8.2	-	-	-	0.1	-	-
Sweden	92.3	-	0.5	-	0.2	0.6	0.1	1.7	0.5	0.1	0.3	1.0	0.3	0.1
United Kingdom	165.2	-	0.3	0.2	0.2	-	-	5.9	0.2	-	0.7	3.3	2.6	0.8
United States	1 068.1	0.4	0.3	0.8	0.2	0.5	-	4.4	1.5	6.5	10.0	19.2	13.7	17.2

Source: Bulletin of World Trade in Engineering Products, 1983 (United Nations publication, Sales No. 85.II.E.11).

Annex V (continued)

Exports and imports of electromedical equipment of selected countries in 1984

(Millions of US dollars)

Exporting country	Total	Bulgaria	Czechoslovakia	German Dem. Republic	Hungary	Poland	Romania	USSR	Yugoslavia	Argentina	Brazil	China	India	Mexico
Czechoslovakia	36.8	0.5	-	6.4	1.5	9.4	0.3	17.2	0.1	-	-	0.6	-	-
France	115.6	-	0.2	0.1	-	0.3	-	0.9	0.1	0.1	1.8	1.7	0.7	2.4
German Dem. Republic	80.0	3.9	8.7	-	5.8	7.9	2.2	45.1	0.4	-	-	1.0	-	-
Germany, Fed. Rep. of	638.8	6.7	6.3	...	2.8	5.8	0.3	16.2	8.4	1.2	6.7	14.2	5.1	3.3
Hungary	23.6	0.5	1.7	0.7	-	4.4	0.6	10.7	-	-	-	1.6	-	1.4
Japan	495.7	0.1	-	-	-	-	-	3.6	-	1.3	0.9	84.8	8.3	-
Netherlands	296.4	0.2	0.9	0.8	0.3	1.0	-	1.3	2.3	0.9	1.2	3.7	4.1	0.2
Poland	12.8	0.1	2.8	0.6	0.8	-	-	8.5	-	-	-	-	-	-
Sweden	84.7	0.2	0.6	-	0.5	0.5	-	2.4	0.7	-	0.6	0.5	0.3	-
United Kingdom	151.8	0.1	0.3	-	-	0.3	-	0.9	0.5	-	0.2	2.7	1.2	-
United States	1 082.6	0.1	0.1	0.1	0.1	1.1	-	2.5	1.1	5.7	6.4	27.7	8.5	22.9

Source: Bulletin of World Trade in Engineering Products, 1984 (United Nations publication, Sales No. 86.II.E.10).

ECE WORKING PARTY ON ENGINEERING
INDUSTRIES AND AUTOMATION

QUESTIONNAIRE FOR THE ECE STUDY ON CURRENT DEVELOPMENTS AND TRENDS
IN MEDICAL EQUIPMENT WITH EMPHASIS ON DIGITAL IMAGE PROCESSING

National report

1. DIGITAL IMAGE PROCESSING (DIP) IN HEALTH CARE

1.1 Statistical information on the number of medical imaging devices in use

DIP device	Number of units installed in/ total in use by						No. of examin- ations 1985
	1980		1985		1990 (estimate)		
	inst.	total in use	inst.	total in use	inst.	total in use	
X-ray							
Film-based X-ray							
Fluoroscopic X-ray							
Digital X-ray							
Digital subtraction angiography							
CT scanner							
Nuclear medicine							
Gamma camera							
Single photon emission tomography							
Positron emission tomograph							
MRI							
Magnetic resonance imaging devices							
Ultrasound							
Ultrasound devices							
PACS							
Picture archiving and communication systems							
Diagnostic work- station							

1.2 <u>Safety legislation and standards for DIP</u>
    (give a short summary with references)

1.3 <u>Adopted policies for purchasing, use etc. of DIP technology</u>
    (give a short summary with references)

1.4 <u>Any public evaluations available on cost-effectiveness, technology
    assessments, etc. of DIP devices</u>
    (give a short summary with references)

2. DIP INDUSTRY

2.1 <u>Statistical information about the companies active in the DIP field</u>

Company	List of main products in DIP	Turnover (currency) in DIP	total	Markets home/export (% / %)	list of countries

2.2 <u>Brief company profiles in verbatim</u>
    (give a short summary concerning ownership, traditions in the DIP
    field/health care/related fields, R and D investment as a percentage of
    turnover, R and D partnerships with research institutes and clinical
    medicine, etc.).

3. RESEARCH AND DEVELOPMENT (R AND D) IN MEDICAL DIP

3.1 <u>Ongoing government supported R and D and university-based R and D
    activities closely related to the application of DIP in medicine</u>
    (give a short summary with references)

3.2 <u>International R and D co-operation in DIP</u>
    (give a short summary with references)

3.3 <u>Amount of public funding available for DIP</u>
    (give a short summary with references)

4. ADDITIONAL COMMENTS

Country:

QUESTIONNAIRE FOR THE ECE STUDY ON DIGITAL IMAGING
IN HEALTH CARE

National report

Purpose of this questionnaire

To obtain national data about the level of diffusion of imaging modalities, about the image generation and processing equipment industry and about research in this field.

For this reason data is collected on both the conventional imaging modalities, such as film-based and fluoroscopic X-ray, and on newer ones, such as MRI devices.

1. IMAGE GENERATION AND PROCESSING IN HEALTH CARE

1.1 Statistical information on the number of medical imaging devices in use

Device type	Number of units in use in			Number of examinations
	1980	1985	1990 (est.)	1985 d/
X-ray				
Film-based X-ray a/				
Fluoroscopic X-ray b/				
Digital subtraction angiography				
CT scanner				
Nuclear medicine				
Gamma camera				
Single photon emission tomography				
Positron emission tomograph				
MRI				
Magnetic resonance imaging devices				
Ultrasound				
Ultrasound imaging devices c/				
PACS				
Picture archiving and communication systems				
Diagnostic work-station				

For footnotes, see next page.

a/ Film-based X-ray includes conventional X-ray equipment where the images are acquired with the use of X-ray film, e.g. for thorax and mammographic examinations. Excluded is dental X-ray equipment.

b/ Fluoroscopic X-ray comprises an X-ray generator assembly equipped with an image-intensifying tube for image acquisition and a fluoroscopic screen, TV monitor and video or a cine camera for image display and storage.

c/ Ultrasound imaging devices comprise systems that produce images either in analogue or digital form. They exclude devices used solely for blood flow studies, e.g. Doppler ultrasound.

d/ An X-ray examination results in a number of exposures (images).

SELECTED BIBLIOGRAPHY

1.   TECHNOLOGY ASSESSMENTS, COST-EFFECTIVENESS STUDIES, ETC.

Health care - general:
Measuring Health Care 1960-1983; Expenditure, Costs and Performance,
OECD Social Policy Studies No.2, Paris, 1985.

DIP:
Gregory A. Baxes. Digital Image Processing; Prentice Hall, Englewood Cliffs
(NJ), 1984.

H. Sochurek. "Medicine's new vision". National Geographic, vol.171, No.1,
pp. 2-41, January 1987.

Evaluation guidelines:
M.F. Drummond, et al. Guidelines for the Evaluation of Digital Diagnostic
Imaging Equipment or Units, Department of Radiology, McMaster University,
Hamilton, Ontario, July 1983.

DA:
Menken, M., et al. The Cost Effectiveness of Digital Subtraction Angiography
in the Diagnosis of Cerebrovascular Disease (Health Technology Case Study 3V,
OTA-HCS-34, Washington, DC. US Congress, Office of Technology Assessment,
May 1985.

CT:
Policy Implications of the Computed Tomography (CT) Scanner: An Update.
Office of Technology Assessment, US Congress, OTA-BP-H.8, January 1981.

MRI:
Health Technology Case Study 27. Nuclear Magnetic Resonance Imaging
Technology: A Clinical, Industrial and Policy Analysis. Washington, DC.
US Congress Office of Technology Assessment, OTA-HCS-27, September 1984.

PACS:
DIN Report: Functional Requirements for a Hospital-based Digital Imaging
Network and Picture Archiving and Communication Prototype System, Washington,
April 1985.

2.   JOURNALS

Journal on Health Technology Assessment

Biomedical Business International

Diagnostic Imaging

Medical Physics

Physics in Medicine and Biology

Journal of Computer Assisted Tomography

Radiology

International Journal of Radiation, Oncology, Biology, Physics

Journal of Nuclear Medicine

British Journal of Radiology

Neuroradiology

Journal of Clinical Ultrasound

Computer Programs in Biomedicine

3. CONFERENCES (PROCEEDINGS)

CAR   Biannual, Computer Assisted Radiology, next 1-4 July 1987,
                  Berlin

MEDINFO   Tri-annual, sponsored by IFIP, last in October 1986,
                  Washington, DC, United States of America, next Peking, China,
                  in 1989

MIE   Biannual, sponsored by EFMI, next 21-25 September 1987, Rome

ICMBE and ICMP   Tri-annual, sponsored jointly by IFMBE and IOMP, next 1988,
                  San Antonio, United States of America, 1991, Kyoto, Japan

WCUMB   Tri-annual, sponsored by WFUMB, next 1988

Note: Information on the forthcoming PACS-related conference may be obtained
directly from the EuroPACS secretariat. [83]

Annex IX

SELECTED TERMINOLOGY

Angiography: A fluoroscopic examination for the imaging of blood vessels where a contrast medium is injected into the arteries.

Doppler device: A radar-like device used to measure the velocity of blood flow through the arteries.

Dynamic range: The range available for expressing the value of a pixel element in bits, where a range of n bits indicates that there are 2^n possible values to that element.

Fluoroscopy: Imaging of the body with X-rays. The image is acquired using an image intensifier that displays the image on a screen. Cine or video camera can be connected to the output screen making recording of dynamic phenomena possible.

Image technology: Any operations conducted on images that capture, synthesize, record, reproduce, convert, process, distribute, transmit and display using photographic, electronic, computer or hybrid methods (ISO/IEC).

Ionizing radiation: A form of radiant energy within the electromagnetic spectrum that has the capability of penetrating solid objects and altering the electrical charge of their atoms. High-energy radiation, such as X-rays and gamma rays, is ionizing radiation.

Magnetic field gradient: A magnetic field that increases or decreases in strength in a given direction along a sample.

Medical technology: The drugs, devices, medical and surgical procedures used in medical care, and the organizational and supportive systems within which such care is provided.

Non-invasive technique: A diagnostic method that does not involve the penetration (by surgery or hypodermic needle) of the skin.

Pixel: Picture element, used to express the amount of picture elements in an image.

Radio-frequency waves: Low-energy, electromagnetic waves.

Resonance: The oscillation of nuclei between higher and lower energy levels as radio-frequency energy is applied and withdrawn.

Sensitivity: The number of positive test results divided by the number of patients that actually have the disease.

<u>Spatial resolution</u>: The extent to which two adjacent structures can be distinguished.

<u>Specificity</u>: The number of negative test results divided by the number of patients that actually have the disease.

<u>Tesla</u>: Unit used for expressing the strength of magnetic fields.

<u>Tomographic scan</u>: The image of an individual slice or plane.

REFERENCES

[1]   ECE Seminar on Innovation in Biomedical Equipment (Budapest, Hungary,
        2-6 May 1983), report of the Seminar (ECE document ENG.AUT/SEM.2/3).

[2]   ECE Working Party on Engineering Industries and Automation,
        fourth session, 7-9 March 1984 (ECE/ENG.AUT/14).

[3]   Preliminary draft outline for a study on innovation in biomedical
        equipment, Note by the ECE secretariat (report ENG.AUT/AC.9/R.1).

[4]   First ad hoc Meeting for the present study, held at Geneva on
        15-16 November 1984 (report ENG.AUT/AC.9/2).

[5]   ECE Working Party on Engineering Industries and Automation,
        fifth session, 27 February-1 March 1985 (report ECE/ENG.AUT/21).

[6]   ECE Working Party on Engineering Industries and Automation,
        sixth session, 19-21 March 1986 (report ECE/ENG.AUT/24).

[7]   Progress report on the present Study, Note by the ECE secretariat
        (ENG.AUT/R.39).

[8]   Second ad hoc Meeting for the present Study, held at Geneva from
        30 June to 2 July 1986 (report ENG.AUT/AC.9/4).

[9]   ECE Seminar on Automation Means in Preventive Medicine '87 (Piestany,
        Czechoslovakia, 28 September-2 October 1987), Information Notice No. 1
        for the Seminar (ENG.AUT/SEM.6/1).

[10]   Safety of Electromedical Equipment. Part 1 - General Requirements for
        Safety, IEC Publication 601-1, Geneva, first edition, 1977.

[11]   Health-care technologies comprise all diagnostic and therapeutic
        procedures, including equipment and devices and other technologies that
        support these procedures.

[12]   Policy implications of the computed tomography (CT) scanner. An
        Update. Office of Technology Assessment, US Congress. OTA-BP-H-8,
        January 1981, p.9.

[13]   Computerized tomography in Sweden. Costs and effects. SPRI,
        Stockholm, December 1981. In Swedish.

[14]   For information contact: WHO Regional Office for Europe, Office for
        Appropriate Technology for Health, Copenhagen.

[15]   The use of technology in the care of the elderly and the disabled:
        tools for living. Ed. by Jean Bray and Sheila Wright. London, 1980.

[16]   IEC Publication 513. Geneva, 1976 and IEC Publication 601-1,
        sub-clause 6.8. Geneva, 1977.

[17] Quality assurance measurements in diagnostic radiology. Hospital Physicists' Association. London, report No.29, 1979.

[18] "Computer guides brain surgeon", Electronics Week, 25 March 1985, pp.19-20.

[19] A. Harman. Portable Image Processing, Systems International, August 1986.

[20] Technical Specifications for the X-ray Apparatus to be used in a Basic Radiological System. World Health Organization. RAD 85/1, 1985.

[21] Fuji Photo Film Co. Ltd., Japan, marketing brochures.

[22] M. Menken, et al. The Cost Effectiveness of Digital Subtraction Angiography in the Diagnosis of Cerebrovascular Disease (Health Technology Case Study 3V, OTA-HCS-34), Washington, DC: US Congress, Office of Technology Assessment, May 1985.

[23] Digital angiography. Technology, medicine, economy, planning and market review; SPRI report 189:2, Stockholm, March 1985.

[24] Office of Technology Assessment, US Congress, Policy Implications of the Computed Tomography (CT) Scanner, GPO Stock No.052-003-00565-4, Washington, DC. US Governmental Printing Office, August 1978.

[25] Computerized tomography in Sweden. Costs and effects. SPRI, Stockholm, December 1981. In Swedish.

[26] Policy implications of the computed tomography (CT) scanner. An Update. Office of Technology Assessment, US Congress. OTA-BP-H-8, January 1981, p.9.

[27] Clinica, 2 September, 1983.

[28] Office of Technology Assessment, US Congress, Policy Implications of the Computed Tomography (CT) Scanner, GPO Stock No.052-003-00565-4, Washington, DC. US Government Printing Office, August 1978, p.30.

[29] Ibid., p.32.

[30] Ibid., p.33.

[31] Computerized tomography in Sweden. Costs and effects. SPRI, Stockholm, December 1981. In Swedish.

[32] Future use of new imaging technologies in developing countries. WHO, Technical Report Series 723, Geneva, 1985.

[33] H. Dahlin, et al. User requirements on CT-based computed dose planning systems in radiation therapy. Acta Radiologica Oncology, 22, 1983, Fasc. 5, pp.398-415.

[34] H.N. Wagner. <u>1984 SNM Meeting Highlights</u>. Society of Nuclear Medicine, Newsletter, September 1984.

[35] B. Vinocur. "Progress comes slowly in radiopharmaceuticals". <u>Diagnostic Imaging</u>, August 1985, pp.60-65.

[36] <u>Performance requirements of scintillation cameras</u>. National Electrical Manufacturers Association (NEMA), Washington, DC, Standards publication No. NU 1-1980.

[37] G.L. Brownell, <u>et al</u>. <u>The future of positron imaging</u>.

[38] M.E. Phelps and T.C. Mazziotta. "Positron emission tomography: human brain function and biochemistry". <u>Science</u>, vol.228, 1985, p.799.

[39] B. Vinocur. "Progress comes slowly in radiopharmaceuticals". <u>Diagnostic Imaging</u>, August 1985, pp.60-65.

[40] <u>Diagnostic Ultrasound Imaging in Pregnancy</u>. National Institute of Health. Consensus Development Conference. Consensus Statement, Vol.5, No.1, 1984.

[41] <u>Methods of measuring the performance of ultrasonic pulse-echo diagnostic equipment</u>, IEC publication 854 - based on document 29D(Central Office)16, Geneva, April 1986.

[42] IEC/SC 29D - medical equipment subjects under consideration by various working groups (WG):

  - Measurement of output dental units - WG 7
  - Measurement of output surgical units - WG 7
  - Measurement and characterization of ultrasonic fields generated by medical ultrasonic equipment using hydrophones in the range 0.5 to 15 MHz - WG 8
  - Pulse-echo diagnostic equipment - WG 9
  - Methods of measurement of the performance of ultrasonic diagnostic equipment - WG 10
  - Labelling requirements for patient acoustic exposure from medical ultrasound equipment for <u>in vivo</u> use - WG 12
  - Exposure and dosimetric standard for medical ultrasound equipment - WG 12
  - Ultrasonic Doppler fetal heart beat detector - 29D(Sec.)30

[43] Ultrasound medical diagnostic equipment (nomenclature of indicators); Standard GOST 4.389-85, USSR State Committee for Standards, Moscow, 1986.

[44] Ultrasonic diagnosis. Principles, economy, choice of equipment. SPRI, Stockholm, September 1980. In Swedish.

[45] <u>Future use of new imaging technologies in developing countries</u>. WHO, Technical Report Series 723, Geneva, 1985.

[46]   Health Technology Case Study 27. Nuclear Magnetic Resonance Imaging
        Technology: A Clinical, Industrial and Policy Analysis.
        Washington, DC. US Congress Office of Technology Assessment,
        OTA-HCS-27, September 1984, p.3.

[47]   High Technology, August 1984, pp.72-73.

[48]   Health Technology Case Study 27. Nuclear Magnetic Resonance Imaging
        Technology: A Clinical, Industrial and Policy Analysis.
        Washington, DC. US Congress Office of Technology Assessment,
        OTA-HCS-27, September 1984, pp.64 and 65.

[49]   R.G. Evens, et al. "Economic and utilization analysis of magnetic
        resonance imaging units in the United States in 1985",
        Am. J. Roentgenology, vol.145, 1985, pp.393-398.

[50]   Magnetic Resonance Imaging, SPRI report 206, Stockholm. In Swedish.

[51]   Health Technology Case Study 27. Nuclear Magnetic Resonance Imaging
        Technology: A Clinical, Industrial and Policy Analysis.
        Washington, DC. US Congress Office of Technology Assessment,
        OTA-HCS-27, September 1984, p.30.

[52]   M. Kuwahara and S. Eiho. "Left ventricular image processing".
        Proceedings of XIV ICMBE and VII ICMP, Espoo, Finland, 11-16 August
        1985, pp.244-247.

[53]   Based on a contribution by E. Bengtsson from IMTEC-Image Technology AB,
        Uppsala, Sweden.

[54]   L. Ferrari and M. Zoeller. "Existing and future capabilities in
        instrumentation magnetic recording". In A. Duerinckx (Ed.). PACS I,
        Proceedings of SPIE. vol.318, 1982, pp.56-59.

[55]   G.G. Cox, et al. "Digital image management". Med. Instrum. 20 (1986),
        pp.208-219.

[56]   M. Iio. "A planned system for Communication and Digital Storage in
        Radiology". Internal report Dept. of Radiology, Faculty of Medicine,
        University of Tokyo, 1985.

[57)   Electronic Business, March 1984, p.164.

[58]   Biomedical Business International, vol.VIII, p.153.

[59]   Ibid., vol.VII, p.117.

[60]   Health Technology Case Study 27. Nuclear Magnetic Resonance Imaging
        Technology: A Clinical, Industrial and Policy Analysis.
        Washington, DC. US Congress Office of Technology Assessment,
        OTA-HCS-27, September 1984, pp.55-56.

[61]   Ibid., p.31.

[62]   ISO technical committees (TC) active in fields related to DI:

         - TC36 - Cinematography
         - TC42 - Photography
         - TC97 - Information processing systems
         - TC130 - Graphic technology
         - TC170 - Micrographics

         For more details see ISO Memento 1985, issued by the ISO central
         secretariat, 1 rue de Varembé, Case postale 56, CH-1211 Geneva 20,
         Switzerland.

         IEC technical committees (TC) and sub-committees (SC) active in fields
         related to DI:

         - TC29 - Electroacoustics
            - SC29D - Ultrasonics

         - TC45 - Nuclear instrumentation
            - SC45B - Radiation protection instrumentation

         - TC62 - Electrical equipment in medical practice
            - SC62A - Common aspects of electrical equipment used in medical
                      practice

            - SC62B - X-ray equipment operating up to 400 kV and accessories

            - SC62C - High-energy radiation equipment and equipment for
                      nuclear medicine

            - SC62D - Electromedical equipment

         - TC83 - Information technology equipment

         For more details see IEC 1986 Yearbook (World standards for electrical
         and electronic engineering), issued by the IEC central office, 3 rue de
         Varembé, CH-1211 Geneva 20, Switzerland.

[63]   IEC particular requirements for the safety of ultrasonic medical
         diagnostic equipment, SC62D (Secretariat) 31.

[64]   Health Technology Case Study 27. Nuclear Magnetic Resonance Imaging
         Technology: A Clinical, Industrial and Policy Analysis.
         Washington, DC. US Congress Office of Technology Assessment,
         OTA-HCS-27, September 1984, p.26.

[65]   M.F. Drummond, et al. Guidelines for the Evaluation of Digital
         Diagnostic Imaging Equipment or Units, Department of Radiology,
         McMaster University, Hamilton, Ontario. July 1983.

[66]   Technical Specifications for the X-ray Apparatus to be used in a Basic
         Radiological System. World Health Organization. RAD 85/1, 1985.

[67]   Health Technology Case Study 27. Nuclear Magnetic Resonance Imaging
        Technology: A Clinical, Industrial and Policy Analysis.
        Washington, DC. US Congress Office of Technology Assessment,
        OTA-HCS-27, September 1984, p.60.

[68]   J. Polakova, J. Gëro. Digital X-ray Processing Based on the Use of
        Equipment Available on Czechoslovakia, CHIRANA-VUZT, Brno, 1984. In
        Czech.

[69]   F. Drastich, K. Jan, J. Kubak. Digital Processing of X-ray Images,
        VUT-FET, Brno, 1984. In Czech.

[70]   M. Sobotka, L. Sorm. Basic Principles of Digital Image Processing,
        TESLA-VUST, Prague, 1985. In Czech.

[71]   C. Greger. Study on the Use of Available Equipment for Digitization of
        X-ray Images. CHIRANA-VUZT, Brno, 1985. In Czech.

[72]   Y. Bizais, et al. The DIMI system philosophy and state of
        development; internal report, Centre Hospitalier Régional, Nantes.

[73]   R. Renoulin, et al. Le projet SIRENE (in French). Paper prepared for
        the ECE Seminar on Automation Means on Preventive Medicine '87 –
        see [9].

[74]   "French Radiology". Diagnostic Imaging International, October 1986.

[75]   W. Bautz and J. Kolbe. Is PACS feasible for a Major Department of
        Radiology, Digit. Bilddiagn. 6(1986)43-48. In German.

[76]   T. Wendler. "Workstation design for the interactive interpretation of
        medical images". Proceedings XIV ICMBE and VII ICMP, Espoo, Finland,
        11-16 August 1985, pp.223-226.

[77]   IEC Publication 788: Medical Radiology-Terminology, IEC, Geneva, 1984.

[78]   Basic quality control in diagnostic radiology. AAPM Report 4,
        Chicago, 1978.

[79]   Performance requirements of scintillation cameras. National Electrical
        Manufacturers Association (NEMA), Washington, DC, Standards
        publication No.NU1-1980.

[80]   Health Technology Case Study 27. Nuclear Magnetic Resonance Imaging
        Technology: A Clinical, Industrial and Policy Analysis.
        Washington, DC. US Congress Office of Technology Assessment,
        OTA-HCS-27, September 1984, p.49.

[81]   CART news, No.1-4. Available from CART secretariat,
        Bildbehandlingseentrum, Box 1704, S-75147 Uppsala, Sweden.

[82]   BAZIS in Leiden together with Philips and the University Hospital in
        Utrecht are planning to carry out an evaluation of the Marcom fully
        digital imaging and PAC system produced by Philips (IMAGIS project).

[83]   EuroPACS Newsletter: Editor J.P.J. de Valk, BAZIS-Leiden University
        Hospital, AZL-Building 50, Rijnsburgerweg 10, 2333 AA Leiden
        (The Netherlands).

[84]   J.P.J. de Valk, et al. "PACS reviewed: Possible and Coming Soon?"
        MEDINFO-86 Proceedings, North-Holland, 1986.

ECE PUBLICATIONS ON ENGINEERING INDUSTRIES AND AUTOMATION

Sales publications */

Recent Trends in Flexible Manufacturing (ECE/ENG.AUT/22),
Sales No.E.85.II.E.35, New York, 1986. $33.00.

Production and Use of Industrial Robots (ECE/ENG.AUT/15),
Sales No.E.84.II.E.33, New York, 1985. $25.00.

Measures for Improving Engineering Equipment with a view to More Effective
Energy Use (ECE/ENG.AUT/16), Sales No.E.84.II.E.25, New York, 1984. $16.50.

Engineering Equipment and Automation Means for Waste-Water Management in ECE
Countries, vols.I and II (ECE/ENG.AUT/18), Sales Nos.E.84.II.E.13 and
E.84.II.E.23, New York, 1984. $12.50 (vol.I) and $8.50 (vol.II).

Techno-Economic Aspects of the International Division of Labour in the
Automotive Industry (ECE/ENG.AUT/11), Sales No.E.83.II.E.14, New York, 1983.
$23.00.

Development of Airborne Equipment to Intensify World Food Production
(ECE/ENG.AUT/4), Sales No.E.81.E.24, New York, 1981. $16.00.

Annual Reviews of Engineering Industries and Automation

1983-1984, vols.I and II (ECE/ENG.AUT/19), Sales No.E.85.II.E.43.
$27.00 (vols.I and II).
1982 (ECE/ENG.AUT/17), Sales No.E.84.II.E.12. $11.00.
1981 (ECE/ENG.AUT/10), Sales No.E.83.II.E.20. $11.00.
1980 (ECE/ENG.AUT/7),   Sales No.E.82.II.E.18. $13.50.
1979 (ECE/ENG.AUT/3),   Sales No.E.81.II.E.16. $8.00.

Bulletins of Statistics on World Trade in Engineering Products

1984, Sales No.E/F/R.86.II.E.10. $38.00.
1983, Sales No.E/F/R.85.II.E.11. $35.00.
1982, Sales No.E/F/R.84.II.E.5. $38.00.
1981, Sales No.E/F/R.83.II.E.8. $38.00.
1980, Sales No.E/F/R.82.II.E.5. $26.00.
1979, Sales No.E/F/R.81.II.E.13. $26.00.

---

*/ Sales publications and documents out of print may be requested in the
form of microfiches.

Price per microfiche $1.65; printed on paper $0.15 per page.

Documents issued in mimeograph form

Reports of Seminars held under the auspices of the ECE Working Party on Engineering Industries and Automation as from 1981:

Seminar on Industrial Robotics '86 - International Experience, Developments and Applications, Brno, Czechoslovakia, 24-28 February 1986 (ENG.AUT/SEM.5/4).

Seminar on the Development and Use of Powder Metallurgy in Engineering Industries, Minsk, Byelorussian SSR, 25-29 March 1985 (ENG.AUT/SEM.4/3).

Seminar on Flexible Manufacturing Systems: Design and Applications, Sofia, Bulgaria, 24-28 September 1984 (ENG.AUT/SEM.3/4).

Seminar on Innovation in Biomedical Equipment, Budapest, Hungary, 2-6 May 1983 (ENG.AUT/SEM.2/3).

Seminar on Present Use and Prospects for Precision Measuring Instruments in Engineering Industries, Dresden, German Democratic Republic, 20-24 September 1982 (ENG.AUT/SEM.1/3).

Seminar on Automation of Assembly in Engineering Industries, Geneva, Switzerland, 22-25 September 1981 (AUTOMAT/SEM.8/3).